what's a lemon squeezer doing in my vagina?

A MEMOIR OF INFERTILITY

ROHINI S. RAJAGOPAL

EBURY
PRESS

An imprint of Penguin Random House

EBURY PRESS

USA | Canada | UK | Ireland | Australia
New Zealand | India | South Africa | China

Ebury Press is part of the Penguin Random House group of companies
whose addresses can be found at global.penguinrandomhouse.com

Published by Penguin Random House India Pvt. Ltd
7th Floor, Infinity Tower C, DLF Cyber City,
Gurgaon 122 002, Haryana, India

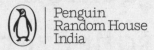

First published in Ebury Press by Penguin Random House India 2021

10 9 8 7 6 5 4 3 2 1

All the medical and scientific information presented in this book is based on the
author's layperson understanding of infertility and from her own experience of
infertility treatment. Most of it has been sourced from publicly available websites
on the Internet with due acknowledgement. It is meant to contextualize and clarify
the emotional and physical journey that the author went through. It is in no way
meant to serve as expert advice on the topic or as a substitute for consultation with
a qualified medical professional.

The author has narrated the experiences captured in this book to the best of her
recollection. Scenes and dialogue have been recreated. Names of people and places
have been changed or left out altogether and physical characteristics and details
modified to protect privacy, except where explicit permission has been obtained.

The views and opinions expressed in this book are the author's own and the facts
are as reported by her which have been verified to the extent possible, and the
publishers are not in any way liable for the same.

ISBN 9780143452003

Typeset in Minion Pro by Manipal Technologies Limited, Manipal
Printed at Thomson Press India Ltd, New Delhi

www.penguin.co.in

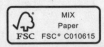

EBURY PRESS

WHAT'S A LEMON SQUEEZER
DOING IN MY VAGINA?

Rohini S. Rajagopal was leading a fairly humdrum life in Bangalore when an encounter with infertility stopped her in her tracks. In a temporary suspension of good sense, she quit her well-paying, flexible-hours job to write this book that narrates her journey from infertility to motherhood. But for her current penury, she has no regrets about that move.

She has a master's degree in English (media and communication). Her special talents include fitting dishes inside overfilled refrigerators and taking three-hour-long afternoon naps without the slightest trace of guilt. You can find her on Instagram at rajagopal.rohini.

For Achan

Contents

Introduction

When I completed the first trimester of my pregnancy I went on a calling binge, ringing up close friends and family to share the good news. Most people said, 'Congratulations! We are happy for you.' Or something to that effect. My husband and I had been married for seven years by then, and they must have felt this call was a long time coming. Only one relative asked, 'Was it IVF?' The 'inordinate delay' must have tipped her off.

'No,' I lied.

'Not IVF? You didn't seek *any* treatment?' she sounded perplexed.

'No, nothing,' I insisted, now cornered by the first lie.

'It happened *naturally*?' she persisted.

'Yes,' I mumbled, wishing this interrogation would just end.

'Okay, then. Congratulations!' she replied mutedly, still unbelieving. I hurriedly put the phone down and hoped this would never come up again.

That lie was a reflex reaction to a blatant, aggressive line of questioning. In that fight-or-flight moment, my instinct was abject denial. I knew her question came from a place of curiosity, from the need to reconfirm a suspicion. *I always knew it. It had to be IVF.* My self-preservation instincts kicked in and I signed out of that conversation. But why did I feel apprehended? As if I had been caught in an act of wrongdoing, as if I had to answer for some dishonourable deed? It was the staunch belief in my own shame. The shame I felt towards myself, my body and my reproductive system, which required such a lengthy, convoluted and 'artificial' intervention to have something as seemingly simple and ubiquitous as a baby.

It's been a long and difficult walk from *that* conversation to *this* book. From being fully convinced about my own 'defectiveness' and the consequent shame, to shedding such convictions, layer after layer; from disclaiming my history to laying bare the secrets of the hospital folder stashed in the drawers underneath our bed. But I am glad that I started the journey to owning the biggest truth of my life.

This book talks about my five-year battle with infertility. I never thought it would take so long to have a baby or that it would cost us the kind of emotional, physical and financial resources it did. When I found success I promised myself that I would share my story. I felt obligated to those who were breaking the Internet every day looking for a few kilobytes of hope. But once I began writing my story I realized that it is one worth telling—happy ending or not—because it throws at least a chink of light on the world of infertility, a world eclipsed by shame, stigma and silence.

While this book documents the series of medical procedures that I underwent, it also speaks about the fear, sorrow, insecurity, desperation, societal pressures and self-expectations that took their toll on my marriage, my psyche and my life. I came to recognize not only how *far* modern medicine can go but also that it can go only *this* far. I ended up questioning my own desire to have a child and the notion of 'infertility' itself. I must warn you that though this is a story of inspiration, it is also a story of repeated failures. It is a story about the transformative powers of reproductive science, but it is also a story about the ugliness of infertility treatment. It is a story about birth, but it is also a story about death, multiple deaths.

The second impulse to tell the story came from a more personal and territorial space. My mother-in-law thinks my son is the answer to her dogged prayers, pujas and offerings. My mother always talks about how intense her longing was to be a grandmother and how much the delay in becoming one hurt. She never missed an opportunity to tell guests who came to see my newborn son that he was born after eight long years of marriage, as if the wait was hers. Elderly aunts and uncles in the family use my story like a cautionary tale for newly-weds: 'Look, they waited so long and see what happened. Have a baby as soon as you can.' But none of these accounts talks about me or my suffering. They don't even use words such as 'infertility'.[1] They are versions of my tale told from a sanitized

---

[1] I myself started using the term 'infertility' to describe my difficulties with conception only after I began this book. Until then it was a dirty secret and I only wished to get past 'infertility' and pretend like it never happened. But both, the act of writing and using the term 'infertility', opened the doors to acceptability and validation. Infertility was clearly defined in reproductive medicine. There was cognizance of the physical and psychological suffering it caused. There were technologies, treatments and support groups for healing. There were personal essays and memoirs from fellow travellers. The word offered me the bridge to connect with a larger mass of people travelling the same road. My suffering was real,

and deodorized distance, situating this story purely in the realm of faith, healing and traditional wisdom. After all, who wants to hear the sordid tales of my vagina, cervical mucus and menstrual blood? This book is an attempt to appropriate my own history, to take back my own narrative. Because this is *my* story and *I* am going to tell it. With all the gore and grime.

My third reason for telling this story is that I couldn't sleep for not undoing my own deceit. I waited months, years, but the urge to tell my truth wouldn't die down. It kept bubbling, foaming and frothing inside, making me choke on my own silence. Writing helped release the big woolly knot of unease that was trapped in my chest. Now that I have gathered enough courage to call the knot by its name, give it shape, form and legitimacy of existence, I can finally breathe.

---

palpable, describable and shareable. As someone who was at the receiving end of this 'blemish', I am conscious of the negative cultural meanings attached to this word. Yet, it is an easily recognized and medically defined term and it offers a start to talking about the largely under-acknowledged physical, emotional and medical struggles to achieve parenthood experienced by so many of us.

1

How to Get Pregnant 101

Even though the fertility clinic was only a thirty-minute drive from our house, getting there took almost three months. For both Ranjith and me, it meant admitting that we had failed at something so 'natural', so 'fundamental', something that others like us fulfilled daily, unconsciously, with no medical help or knowledge. It meant overcoming our shame, setting aside our egos and revealing our most naked selves to a stranger.

After days of vacillation, Ranjith and I finally stepped inside a clinic run by a well-known infertility specialist. A dear friend had recommended her name to us. We had booked an appointment with the chief doctor herself, fearing that the visit would be futile if we couldn't meet her. She consulted just two days of the week, and if you didn't specifically request a meeting with her you would wind up with one of the numerous junior doctors who assisted her.

The clinic had an unassuming and almost shabby exterior. It was an old, two-storeyed bungalow repurposed into a mini-hospital, the kind where wooden partitions and glass cabins have been arbitrarily placed in erstwhile living rooms, bedrooms and kitchen. The spartan functionality of its office furniture clashed with the arched hallways, ornate window grills and multi-hued mosaic flooring of the house originally built for loftier purposes. A small, shaded yard led to the main entrance. There was no parking and we left our car in one of the by-lanes nearby. I missed the glitz and swankiness of the all-inclusive corporate hospital, but we were here for the doctor's expertise and not to see posh interiors.

It was 8 a.m. on a Saturday and the reception area was already packed with couples at various stages of treatment. As first-time visitors, we paid the registration fee and went into a consultation room. A bespectacled, presumably junior consultant motioned us to sit down and began inquiring into our condition, reading out queries from a four-page data sheet in her hand and filling it in as the Q&A progressed. There were questions on our medical history, the nature of my menstrual cycle, our lifestyle, hereditary diseases and, of course, the most critical query: how long we had been trying to conceive. That probably did not tick all the boxes, so what followed was a point-by-point probing of our sex life.

'How often do you have intercourse?'

'Once or twice a week.'

'When was the last time you had intercourse?'

'Last Sunday.'

'Have you experienced any sexual dysfunction?'

'No.'

'Do you have any history of sexually transmitted diseases?'

'No.'

Our tone was flat and deadpan, betraying none of the unease we felt, as if it were routine to discuss the schedule and specifications of our sex life. Of course, only I spoke. Ranjith leaned back in his chair, arms folded across his chest, and uttered a syllable or two when a question was specifically directed at him. He had come there only for me.

Once the patient history form was filled up the doctor said she would have to examine me and pointed to a bed in the same room. I knew what was coming and didn't look forward to it, but agreed obediently. Removing my shoes, I stepped on a two-rung stool and climbed onto the steel examination table while she drew a curtain around it.

'Please remove your pyjamas,' she ordered.

I loosened the knot of my salwar, pulled it down along with my underwear and lay down on my back. She wore her gloves, dipped her index and middle fingers in jelly and inserted them inside my vagina, feeling the contours of my insides in rough, rapid moves. I held my breath, interlocked my fingers tightly and focused unblinkingly on the ceiling.

After a few seconds she noted, 'There is nothing anatomically wrong with your body.'

'Hmm,' I exhaled. The only thing I cared for was the departure of the groping fingers and restoration of dignity to my half-naked self.

Back at the table, she handed us a printout that laid down the next steps.

'Please come back once you finish all the tests on this sheet,' she said.

We nodded dutifully and stepped out of the room, our to-do list in hand.

We chose the diagnostics lab first. There were twenty-odd tests to strike off the list—from HIV to blood sugar to the various hormones that govern reproduction. The phlebotomist[1] indicated a student chair and asked me to place my extended arm on the foldable writing pad. He drained several millilitres of my blood into colour-coded vials. I did not fear needles and breathed easily through the prick of skin and tightness of strap. It was certainly easier than offering access to the inner recesses of my vagina. Once I was done, Ranjith sat on the same chair and went through the same motions.

Next was sperm collection. A male technician handed Ranjith a small plastic container with a white label on it. He asked him to make use of a room at the opposite end of the corridor with the sign 'Sample Collection' outside. Ranjith hid the cup in his closed fist and walked into the room. As the door closed I caught a fleeting glimpse of its interiors— peeling walls and a broken chair. I sat on the bench, facing the closed door, trying to block all thoughts. After fifteen minutes he emerged.

The final stop was ultrasound. I was led into a room overpowered by medical equipment and asked to lie down on a long, narrow bed. My salwar and underwear rested on hooks in the bathroom. A chirpy radiologist photographed the insides of my uterus with the transducer, noting down measurements of my ovaries on paper. Once or twice she yelped in delight at the images that appeared on the screen.

'Excellent. A triple lining!' she said.

---

[1] 'A phlebotomist is a person responsible for drawing blood from patients for lab tests, transfusions, or donation.' (Source: Verywellhealth, https://www.verywellhealth.com/what-is-a-phlebotomist-1736261, accessed in October 2020.)

I maintained my breathless silence, again fixated only on when the ultrasound probe would be withdrawn from my vagina.

As soon as Ranjith and I stepped into the clinic, it was as if an invisible wall had emerged to separate us— husband and wife—snapping the lines and wires of marital communication. We walked around the clinic like zombies, taking instructions, undoing zippers, lowering underwear, offering arms for needles . . . It was like a spontaneous, self-imposed blockade. We resisted processing the happenings around us. We resisted conversation. We resisted each other's eyes even, each feeling sickeningly guilty that the other had been dragged into such a distasteful setting. We had come in expecting the privacy and safety of a cosy consultation room, but the fertility clinic turned out to be an open parade in which our self-respect and dignity were systematically poked, squeezed and drained out. It was only about one and a half hours later, when the stripping and skinning were complete, that we were ushered into the cabin of the doctor we had come to meet in the first place.

~

In the early years of our marriage, we were trying *not* to get pregnant. It was one of our first promises to each other. No children until we had arranged all the disorderly parts of our lives into neat piles: career, home, and *then*, children.

We got married in Trivandrum (Thiruvananthapuram) in January 2007 in a conventional minimal-fuss Malayalee Nair wedding that lasted all of twelve minutes; polishing off the five thousand dishes on the plantain leaf at the wedding feast took longer. Exactly a week later, Ranjith and I wrapped up our newly-wed duties and boarded an early morning flight to Bangalore. There were no misty eyes or lumpy throats at the airport, where half my family had gathered to see us off. If anything, there was a repressed air of celebration; my mother was relieved that she was finally getting rid of her problem child. She wished Ranjith luck before waving us goodbye.

I didn't mind her palming me off like that because my twenty-five-year-old self was hopping and skipping merrily down the tarmac, eager to get away. As I looked out the aircraft window at the green canopy zooming out below, there was a surge of hope and happiness. We were finally on our own, having secured the sanction to construct a brand-new life, with all its adventures and ordeals.

Ranjith was leaving a marketing role in an IT company in Hyderabad to join a newly founded venture capital (VC) fund in Bangalore. The VC job offered more money, but it also demanded more sweat and blood. Apart from the drudgery of twelve hours in office, there were dinner parties, networking events, panel discussions and media interactions that he had to attend. As he tried to keep up a constant chase paced to the pursuits of start-ups, there was barely enough space in his life for food and sleep, let alone a new wife.

I was working as a copy-editor in an academic publishing house in Hyderabad when I met Ranjith. When we shifted to Bangalore I found that I was all but 'unemployable', given the paucity of publishers there. Desperate for work, I joined the long queues outside the BPOs that dotted the city. They hired in batches of hundreds and sieved candidates principally on one criterion—the ability to read, write and speak in English. After a few misses I found a position in the knowledge management team of a multinational corporation. Only a miniscule percentage of the job had any congruence with my education and experience. Most of it was like learning to speak a foreign language. I had to create and edit web content and reskill myself in website and document management. It was a rude shock to learn there was more to computers than MS Word and Google, especially for someone who came from the paper-and-pencil world of publishing. But I was game; I did not want to spend one more day sitting at home checking my email every five minutes for responses from Naukri.com.

On the first day of my new job, a lanky HR representative met me at the front office of the mammoth glass-and-steel facility. He sat me down in a vacant conference room and dropped a bomb, otherwise known as 'policy'.

'No mobile phones on the floor. They must be stored in metal lockers lined outside our bays. No personal belongings like wallet, purse, either. Same locker for those as well. You can carry a water bottle if you like but if you forget to take it home in the evening the housekeeping staff will throw it away. No dedicated workspace or computer. These must be shared with another team that occupies the same seats at night. No opening windows or raising the blinds. And no one gets a toe past the gates of the facility without the access card, not even the CEO.'

I was speechless. As he escorted me to the floor my team occupied, I felt I was being enlisted for a secret space mission to Mars. I wanted to tell the man that I had randomly circled 'B's on the aptitude test and did not know any maths or science beyond class three. But it was too late for that.

From there it was a long, exacting tussle to come to grips with corporate life. The job itself turned out to be quite simple, once you got past the technical hyperbole, and the people were warm, friendly and ever-ready to help. But the data security rules and requirements were suffocating, it was a ten-hour working day and the commute in the company cabs made it longer.

~

Ours was not a 'love marriage', but it was not entirely an 'arranged marriage' either. Ranjith and I had spent many evenings and nights together in the months that elapsed between our first meeting and our wedding. But living together in the same house made us realize that we had only skimmed the surface of our relationship.

In most ways we were each other's antonyms. I was a fan of cities, revelling in the neon glint and shine of malls and multiplexes. Ranjith was obsessed with the wild outdoors—the more desolate and inaccessible, the better. He loved the company of friends and family and was at ease in any group setting. I hated any gathering of more than three human beings and suffered panic attacks every time I had to attend one of his office parties. I was organized and disciplined, starting and ending the day with numbered lists on post-it notes. He had utter disdain for agendas and timetables, never having made or stuck to a plan in his life. But, like a lot of youngsters, we found our common ground in travel. Every long weekend was spent driving out of town—to the coffee plantations in Coorg, the cave formations of Yana, the beaches in Gokarna, the forests of Wayanad, the ancient temples in Belur and Halebidu . . . we had seen every place worth visiting within a 500 km radius of Bangalore.

I don't remember ever asking myself if I *wanted* to have children. It was taken for granted, like graduating from college. The only question open to debate was *when*. During a workshop on reproductive health in college, an affable forty-something doctor had suggested that married couples wait at least two years before starting a family. Two years to get to know each other. Two years to develop an understanding of each other before letting in the chaos of parenting. I held on to that number, and as we progressed towards it in our own marriage, I believed we could start trying to have a child.

After the initial months of our relationship, the excitement of lovemaking had worn off, to be replaced by the tedium of everyday life. At the end of a busy working day neither of us had the passion or energy to make love. Sex was a weekends-only chore. But I assumed that whenever we wanted we could get our heads down and make a baby. Except for the fact that we kept putting it off. A holiday to the lonely mountains of Ladakh. A high-stakes deal Ranjith was closing at work. The nerve-wracking and seemingly unending labour of buying and furnishing a two-bedroom apartment. All these took precedence.

In the meantime, I climbed up two levels of the corporate ladder and secured a much-coveted laptop. This gave me the flexibility to work from home for fifteen hours in the week. We shifted to our new sixth-floor flat, which was situated close to my workplace and which slashed my commute time to twenty minutes. I learnt to drive a car after conquering many months of paranoia, happily bidding goodbye to company transport. Ranjith also began to find his feet in the booming world of technology, entrepreneurs and investors. We felt the time was just about right to move to the next life stage.

A married friend had told me that the global average time it takes for a woman to get pregnant was seven months. In a healthy couple with no fertility issues it took seven months of trying before the woman got pregnant. There was no such thing as overnight success—making a baby required planning, monitoring and focused effort. So when Ranjith and I decided we were ready to have a baby, I recalled her advice and embarked on 'Project Baby' in all earnest. I started my research on the Internet, trying to understand the correct timing for intercourse, what ovulation is, how to track it using basal body temperature and cervical mucus changes, and so on. I read the 'How to Get Pregnant 101' articles that suggested tips and easy ways to get pregnant fast. I looked up intercourse positions that were most conducive to conception. Armed with all this information, we tried for several months. We even took special holidays devoted to making a baby, away from the rigours of our routine. But month after month I was disappointed to discover that our efforts had not borne fruit.

All around us, friends, cousins and colleagues were getting married and becoming pregnant right away, and we were falling behind. What made us 'cool' initially now made us the odd ones out. Ranjith's sister had her first child the year I got married. I was happy, excited and involved. But when she was pregnant with her second baby I felt horrible. It was supposed to be *my* turn. How could she skip the queue?

Well-meaning friends said, 'Relax, it will happen. You are thinking too much about it. It will happen when it's least expected.'

Older women in the family offered advice, mostly through my mother.

'Are you on top? Don't be.'

'Do you wash yourself immediately after sex? Don't.'

'Try lying down with a pillow under your buttocks after sex.'

Some were critical: 'You waited too long. You should have started trying the very next day after the wedding.'

The questions about 'good news' had started popping up from both sides of the family soon after our marriage. I ignored them. We had other priorities and had no aspirations to have a child. I laughed when a grand-aunt asked, tentatively, if we had started treatment. 'Can we please give sex a try first?' I thought. But slowly, as my own desire for a child began to grow, the questions began to hurt. I felt the sting of each word. I dreaded spending time alone with Ranjith's mother, knowing the topic would invariably surface. She was a gentle, kind and pious woman, but even *she* could not suppress a slight accusatory note when she said, 'What are you doing? Why are you not pregnant yet?'

My mother was more indirect. She hinted at her own longing to have a grandchild. She spoke about how she envied her friends who were already grandmothers. She brought up all the prying questions *she* had to face at the university where she taught, in the bus on the way to work and everywhere else she went, on her daughter's childless status. The message was, 'Can't you see the kind of pressure *I* am under? Get pregnant, please.'

If I felt burdened by their expectations as well as my own, Ranjith seemed unfazed. He was absolutely convinced that we were going to have a baby. He did not want to know or discuss the technicalities of conception and felt I was overthinking a task best left to nature. He maintained that there was nothing wrong with either of us, and in due course we would have a baby.

He liked to say, 'You could become pregnant tomorrow for all you know.'

But that tomorrow was taking its time to come and I was slowly losing the grip on my mind waiting for it.

At weddings and holiday resorts, airports and cinema halls, I looked around for couples who seemed to be our age and did not have children, as a way of validating our experience. It was a relief to know that we were not the *only* ones. Once, on a late-night movie outing, I spotted a young couple in the basement parking lot of a mall. They were getting into the car next to ours. I assumed that they did not have children because I didn't see any around them. My fantasy lasted only a short while before I noticed a pink hospital file in the rear seat of their sedan. It was a pregnancy folder. My heart sank. Even she was pregnant, just not visibly so. This non-pregnant breed was dwindling rapidly.

When you are denied something, your mind grossly overestimates its value. I rejected all the gifts in our lives and dwelled on its single deficiency. Pregnancy was an exclusive club and I wanted to break in. I envied the special treatment and attention a pregnant woman attracted. She is offered the most comfortable chair. Someone is always ready to carry her bags. Everyone checks on her well-being. In fact, her pregnancy, with its highs and lows, is the very topic of conversation. In some ways, pregnancy was more important to me than having the child itself. I was clear-eyed enough to know that there is nothing glamorous about parenting. It meant clutter, drudgery, illness, responsibility, and tying my life-long happiness to someone else's well-being. Pregnancy, in contrast, seemed like a short-lived, light-hearted summer love. I imagined a breezy nine months spent cradling my baby bump and preening in front of the mirror.

With my Bollywood-themed imagination I kept choreographing the different ways in which I would find out that I was pregnant.

Scenario one. I wake up one day to realize that my period is a few days late. There's an unused home pregnancy test lying in the bathroom. I casually open the pack and place two drops of urine to test, just in case I am . . . and guess what? I *am* pregnant. *Great! I wasn't expecting that.*

Scenario two. I am feeling unusually tired and weak in office. I put it down to work pressure and continue plodding along. When I get up to gather my laptop, charger and data cable for yet another meeting, my head starts spinning and I faint to the ground. Colleagues rush me to hospital and, no, it's not brain tumour or blood cancer . . . I am just *pregnant! What a surprise! Who would have thought?*

I tripped on every aspect of pregnancy. How would I break it to Ranjith? What maternity clothes would I buy? Where would we go for our babymoon? Which birthing clinic would I opt for? How long would I go on maternity leave? Every detail was accounted for while I waited impatiently for the two magic lines to appear on the pregnancy test.

Month after month, in the days leading up to my period, I imagined that I was pregnant. I scrutinized every premenstrual symptom (fatigue, lower abdominal pain, backache) and convinced myself that it had worked this time. I googled pregnancy symptoms and matched them with my own. I took 'Am I Pregnant?' pop quizzes that said there was a 55 per cent chance that I was pregnant. Some months I took home pregnancy tests (HPTs), and when they turned out negative I searched for stories of women who had false-negative HPTs. I climbed stairs slowly, avoided bending over and rode gently over speed breakers so as to not cause a miscarriage inadvertently. I ate pregnant, slept pregnant, walked pregnant and talked pregnant. I willed and commanded my body to be pregnant—until my period showed up, sometimes five agonizing days late, raising hopes and then dashing them to the ground. Every month I wept and wailed. Each time it felt like I had miscarried. My mind swung between hope, excitement, anticipation and heartbreaking despair. *How could I mourn the loss of something that didn't even exist?*

Things came to a head when at first the 'global-average-time-to-get-pregnant' milestone whooshed past, and then the 'twelve months of regular intercourse without protection' timeframe defined by fertility medicine. I began considering a visit to a fertility specialist. Even after the thought first made its appearance in my head I shelved it for as long as I could, hoping that I could get away with not making that visit, that somehow I would get pregnant before any intervention was sought. But the gnawing feeling began to grow that something *had* to be done. This was not working out left to ourselves. Ranjith still stuck to his view that 'nothing is wrong'.

I pushed and prodded him.

I reasoned, 'At least let us go and find out. If nothing is wrong, then we can relax and wait for it to happen naturally. But if something is wrong it gives us the chance to rectify it.'

~

Finally, we were face-to face with the senior doctor. She was a tall, stately woman with neatly tied hair, and an air of authority. You could tell she was used to dashing off instructions and having cowering subordinates hurrying to comply.

She glanced through the patient file placed on the desk. She had our history and the ultrasound report; the results of the blood tests and semen sample would take a few more days. The assistant doctor stood behind her shoulder like a schoolgirl waiting for the class teacher to finish checking her homework. We sat in silence, eager for her pearls of fertility wisdom.

After a few minutes she turned to the junior doctor who had prepared the file and placed her finger on a sentence in the document. The young doctor, petrified, peered closely at the document.

'What kind of a sentence is this?' said the senior doctor in a censuring tone. 'This is terrible English.'

The young woman's face went blank. She did not offer a response. She kept her eyes locked on the page, trying to figure out what exactly was wrong.

The chief doctor turned to us and explained, 'Just because you are a doctor does not mean you are above grammar. If Shakespeare saw this, he would be turning in his grave.'

We cringed, half-smiling out of polite necessity, but internally resisting this co-option. We didn't see the aim of shaming the younger doctor in front of us nor the doctor's concern for Shakespeare in the grave.

She concluded that, based on preliminary information, there was nothing wrong. She asked us to come back once the other results came in. She also asked us to plan for a hysterosalpingogram (HSG)[2] before launching into a small pep talk on sex positions.

---

[2] 'Hysterosalpingography is a special x ray using dye to look at the womb (uterus) and fallopian tubes.' (Source: Medline Plus, https://medlineplus. gov/ency/article/003404.htm, accessed in August 2020.)

'See, from what I can tell, your problem must be position. Everything else seems to be fine. I will give you a couple of options. These are ideal for conception.'

She opened a notepad and began to sketch figures to illustrate her point. We both looked at the stick figures, trying to project a studious interest in the lesson. She droned on about postural combinations, gravity and the movement of bodily fluids, stopping just short of a demonstration. But by then nothing was making sense to us. Mentally, both of us had fled that room.

For the entire duration of our visit at the fertility clinic Ranjith's body language screamed, 'What are we doing here?' I must have transmitted the same vibes. We felt like two lost tourists who had turned up at the wrong address. This place wasn't for us. I was twenty-eight years old. Ranjith was thirty-three. In the context of assisted reproduction, we were still very young. We had been trying to conceive for only a year, even though we had been married for over three years. I had a regular menstrual cycle and neither of us had any known health issues or family history of infertility. There was no dying need to put ourselves through the rollers of this wringer.

We couldn't wait to gather the little dignity still left in us and run the hell out of that clinic. We vowed never to come back.

2

Where Action = IUI,
Result = Pregnancy

A few months after that first brush with fertility medicine I received a call from my mother at work. It was unusual for her to call at that time because we had a pre-arranged time to talk every day. Sensing that something was amiss I answered at once. My father had been suffering from various minor ailments over the last six months. A persistent cough. A hoarse and feeble voice due to the cough. Anaemia. Weight loss. By themselves, each of these troubles didn't amount to much, but when put together like pieces in a jigsaw puzzle, they revealed an alarming diagnosis. Amma had called to say that my father was suffering from oesophageal cancer. It had already progressed to stage three by the time it was discovered. The prognosis was grim; doctors gave him anything between six months to one and a half years.

After I disconnected the call I raced to the washroom, closed the door behind me and fell to the ground, unable to withstand the realization that something so ghastly had befallen one of us. The next day I tried to call Achan on the phone and offer words of support, but found that difficult to do with a choking lump in my throat. I couldn't even bring myself to enunciate the 'C' word out loud. It took a week before I clicked on a web browser and googled the disease to understand what lay ahead of us. My foremost thought was: *Why us? Everyone's parents seemed to be happy and healthy. Only my father was dying of cancer.*

Achan started chemotherapy and radiation in the Regional Cancer Centre in Trivandrum, hopeful that it would send the cancer into remission. My brother, Gopal, who lived in Chennai, and I alternated with monthly visits to our city where Amma and Achan lived. Achan's life was swiftly reduced to doctor visits, chemo sessions, blood transfusions and short stints of hospitalization. The coughing and breathlessness worsened. He lost weight, hair, voice, appetite and almost everything that made him the man he was. Day-to-day chores—taking a bath, eating breakfast, or just watching TV—became achievements. He was not new to physical infirmity. He had managed in his quietly dignified manner a range of conditions all his life— diabetes, piles, spondylosis, arthritis and heart disease, each taking turns to act up so that it was a never-ending cycle of managing pain and distress. As children we were conscious of his physical limitations and accepted them as a part of who he was. He couldn't run, sit cross-legged on the floor or horse around with us in the house. We knew about 'hypoglycemia' and the danger it signalled. But these were all relatively minor inconveniences in a life that largely bore the semblance of normalcy. Until cancer came and left no room for negotiation, no room for adapting to or softening or resisting its hold. The disease's vicious arms had him by his throat, taking out his life force one sputtering breath at a time.

Achan never asked me directly about having a baby. Once in a while he checked casually with Amma whether we planned to start a family any time soon. He adored babies and toddlers and was a devoted father when we were that age. His yearning to be a grandfather was palpable to everyone around him. Seeing him now in this enfeebled state, I felt I owed him a grandchild. Maybe he wouldn't live long enough to see the baby, but even the news that I was pregnant would give him a fresh lease of hope.

Two months after his treatment began, a fresh CT scan showed that Achan's cancer had metastasized to the lungs. It had now spread beyond the curative powers of medicine. There was nothing much left to do. We turned to palliative care, administering doses of morphine at regular intervals to relax the lung muscles and allay his respiratory difficulties. The only goal was to stretch whatever little quality of life that remained as close to the end as possible.

One quiet afternoon, I was with him in Trivandrum. He was resting in his bedroom, propped up by pillows. Sheaths of warm sunlight filtered in through the open windows of his room. The murmur of swaying coconut tree fronds had lulled him into a light sleep. I was in my own room reading Llosa's *The Bad Girl* when the doorbell rang. I sprang up and scampered to the door, cursing the ill-timed intrusion. The previous night had been particularly rough and Achan had just settled into a nap; I hoped against hope that the shrill sound hadn't woken him up.

It was the postman who had come to deliver an envelope marked 'Registered Post' for my father.

'He is sleeping right now. I will take this; I am his daughter,' I said curtly, eager to dismiss the khaki-clad man.

'No, madam. This is a passport. I can only hand it over to the addressee,' he insisted.

Achan had always wanted to travel abroad, particularly to Europe. For my father—having grown up in a country that was just shedding its colonial skin, and possessing a literary taste for largely British classics—England topped the chart of his must-see places. He was fascinated by the picture-postcard beauty of the countryside, the cathedrals and palaces steeped in history, the royal family and its ceremonial traditions. He scoffed at the Americans, whom he claimed 'had no civilizational history'. However, with the modest salary of a middle-level bank officer and two children to educate, there was no spare income left for holidays, let alone foreign holidays. Amma and Achan scrimped and skimped, pulling off a tightrope walk month after month. They took bank loans to buy each gadget in the house, Amma's *kashu mala*[1] spent more time in mortgage than in her locker, and increments and bonuses were earmarked for expenses before the money reached their accounts. Their financial struggles eased up only after Gopal and I moved out and became financially independent. This gave them the extra buffer to consider what were earlier deemed extravagances. They signed up for membership in a three-star holiday resort network, upgraded their decades-old Maruti 800 for a Maruti 800 AC and started travelling by third-AC rail coaches. But the foreign holiday was still a distant dream.

---

[1] *Kashu mala* is a necklace made of gold coins. It is a piece of traditional Kerala jewellery.

When Achan was diagnosed with cancer, he was discerning enough to know there wasn't much time left and serenely accepted his fate. He had only one wish—he wanted to visit a foreign country. He had applied for a passport in his thirties in anticipation of a job opportunity in the Middle East but that offer never materialized and his passport lay unused. It remained merely an official document, a piece of legal paper used only as proof of address and identity. The expiry date came and went, and no one noticed. Until neck deep in aggressive cancer therapy, Achan resolved to go on a foreign holiday. Maybe not to England, given the long flight and the bitter cold, but to a more practical and short-flight destination, like Singapore or Dubai. To have his passport stamped just once, to visit a world that lay beyond the bounds of his own city, state and country, to extract a small prize from a life that had been so tight-fisted in dispensing its baubles and trinkets. Achan insisted that Amma get his passport renewed.

At first Amma ignored this demand. It was foolish and a waste of time to chase this potentially useless documentation amid more pressing day-to-day concerns. She was single-handedly providing full-time home care to a terminally ill patient. She drove him to chemo sessions and back, stayed up long hours in the night rubbing his back while he coughed ceaselessly and then woke up early in the morning to make 'health foods' suggested by every stranger who passed by—carrot juice, turmeric milk, vegetable soup, ragi porridge—before rushing to the university, twenty-five kilometres away. Besides, applying for and securing a passport then was a two-three-month-long campaign, especially for one that had expired years ago. To add to the complications, Achan's official name differed slightly from document to document. She would have to find a passport agent to book a name-change advertisement in the newspapers and consolidate the various spellings before even submitting an application. It was an unwanted load on a woman already weighed down by too many duties and emotions. But Achan persisted, and Amma, who was incapable of saying no to anything or anyone for too long, gave in. We were still not sure if the passport would get done in time, but at least the ball had been set rolling.

Achan hobbled his way from the bedroom to the front door, holding his mundu with one hand and placing the palm of his other on the walls for support. He scribbled in the row against his name on the postman's delivery receipt and took the brown envelope. I sensed a fleeting moment's regret in the young messenger's eyes for stirring a frail old man from his sleep and making him tread that distance of ten or twenty footsteps to the threshold. But how was he to know that it was a dying man walking to grasp his dying wish? How was he to know that the two would never meet?

Achan went back to his room and leaned against the window, examining the passport in the sunlight. He flipped the pages, stared at his photograph, verified the details and ordered me to inform Amma, who was at work. When he was done, I took the passport into my hands and did the same things he had.

'Congrats, Acha! Passport *kittiyallo*,' I said, as if this missing booklet had been the only hindrance in his life.

'*Athe*,' he said, and flashed an innocent smile.

We held each other in a tight embrace, feeling powerful and hopeful again. It was one of the happiest days of his ebbing life. A day marked by the celebration of a small success amidst a series of disappointments and failures, a day that reattached a faint layer of normalcy to a life that had become unrecognizable and opened up the thin potential of places to go, people to meet and things to see. Even if it was as glaring as that afternoon sun, it was too little, too late.

In August, a month later, back in Bangalore, I called to wish him on the day of Thiruvonam. Achan feebly uttered, 'Happy Onam' before handing the phone back to Amma, not having the energy to expend on any more words. That was our last conversation. By then his hands and feet had become white and swollen, suggesting renal failure. He had stopped eating and was slipping in and out of consciousness, reminding Amma again and again not to subject him to a ventilator if it came to that. Four days later, on 26 August 2010, about nine months after his diagnosis, he passed away. I was standing in line to board an aircraft to Trivandrum when I got the news. I missed being with him by a couple of hours. He missed having a grandchild by much more. Some distances can never be traversed.

~

Another year had passed. Achan's illness and death had consumed it. I spent two weeks in Trivandrum after the cremation and other last rites, helping Amma move in with her own mother. My grandfather had died a few years earlier and Ammamma was staying alone in a sprawling standalone house, built decades ago. It was neither safe nor convenient for mother and daughter to stay apart while living in the same town. So Amma grudgingly gave up the independence and nostalgia-filled rooms of her own house and moved back in with her eighty-year-old mother. I returned to Bangalore and retraced the rhythms of office, home and weekends. Over time the clouds of gloom parted and light slowly reappeared. Before long, the same-old worries relegated to the background in the interlude began to take centrestage.

We had consulted the fertility specialist more than a year ago. The blood and semen analysis had shown that all values were within range. The physical examination had not identified any incongruities. The HSG had demonstrated that my fallopian tubes were patent. But I was still not pregnant and was about to turn thirty in a few months' time. I was twenty-five when I got married to Ranjith and had assumed that we would spend the first two to three years enjoying the independence of being child-free. Ages twenty-eight to thirty had been allotted for the business of childbirth. That deadline was now approaching and I was keen on rounding this off quickly. Traditional wisdom also suggested that it was best to bear a child or two before reaching that number. Until this juncture, I had met every personal target set for myself and didn't want to fall short of this one.

Achan's passing away also led to some lens-cleaning of my priorities. I began to wonder if life was passing us by in the mad dash between office and home. What was the purpose of all this relentless action? Shouldn't the focal point of our efforts and energies be relationships, family, children? A woman's childbearing years are limited, so shouldn't we be giving precedence to family at this point? My fertility was probably already on the decline.

Ranjith's optimism too had taken a beating and he was no longer sure if baby-making would happen on its own. After all, we had been trying for more than two years now.

I took advantage of the cracks that were beginning to appear in his certitude and asked him if we could re-seek medical help. By now we had somewhat digested the disgust from our first encounter with fertility medicine and decided to give it one more go. But this time we resolved not to return to the same clinic. The last time, we had felt like objects in a factory unit being sent from one assembly line to another. Despite the eminence of the doctor (or because of it), she seemed too removed from her patients and too imperious in her ways. We needed a doctor who would come close enough to establish a personal connection with us and who at the same time would stay distant enough to offer a dispassionate cure.

After reviewing a couple of options we zeroed in on Dr Leela, who consulted in a large multi-speciality hospital. I had met her for a minor gynecological problem a few years ago; she had addressed it promptly then. I felt confident about her competence but was not sure if she had specific expertise in infertility treatment. But we decided to visit her because we both felt comfortable with her personality.

She was reserved, but clear, decisive and crisp when she spoke. She expressed concern but did not allow that concern to descend into moralizing. The clincher for us, however, was the logistical ease in consulting her. The hospital was right opposite my office; I just had to cross the road. One Saturday morning in April 2011, Ranjith and I walked in to meet her with all the reports from the previous clinic, ready to bite the same bullet again.

Dr Leela remembered me. She hadn't changed at all from the last time I met her, three years ago. She was slim, light-skinned and curly-haired. She draped the kind of bright, expensive silk saris that I reserved for weddings of close family. That day too I admired her resplendent pink and blue Kancheepuram. It turned out that she did specialize in infertility and lead an IVF clinic that functioned in a separate building within the same hospital premises.

She was her usual economical self, and the meeting wound up in five or seven minutes.

'I don't want to repeat the tests you have already done. It's only been a year,' she said, after poring through our reports. 'Meet me at the IVF clinic on day two or day three of your period next month and we will get started.'

We nodded our heads and left, making way for the hordes of patients waiting in the outpatient department (OPD).

We had already undergone investigations that showed there were no glaring errors to be fixed. We were flag-bearers of the 'unexplained infertility' syndrome; there was no distinct, identifiable cause for infertility. Perhaps the timing of sexual intercourse was off (after all, there is only a two-to-six-day fertile window every month) or the stress of everyday life was hampering our efforts. It seemed as if a little bit of fine-tuning would see us through, and that fertility medicine would supply that fine-tuning. I thought it would be as clean and quick, straightforward and result-assured as treating a bacterial infection with a five-day course of antibiotics; as thoughtless and snappy as inserting a coin and retrieving candy from a vending machine. A simple, linear equation:

where action = IUI (intrauterine insemination),
result = pregnancy.

My naive confidence assumed that I would meet the 'pregnant-by-thirty' goal easily, give or take a couple of months.

Fertility doctors typically hesitate to intervene and start intrusive procedures unless and until a woman crosses thirty-five years of age or there is a known history of menstruation and fertility troubles. Since neither was true in our case, Dr Leela suggested in the next meeting that we try naturally for a few more months. She offered some pills to boost ovulation while we employed the old-fashioned method to make a baby. I was not enthused by this offer and did not quite buy into the theory of 'natural' cycles. *Why go to an IVF clinic for that?* There was a sense of urgency in me. I felt more inclined towards decisive, goal-oriented medical action, not wishy-washy, half-naturopathy, half-allopathy measures.

'Can we give IUI a try?' I asked gingerly.

By now I had devoured the Internet on assisted reproductive technologies (ART) and believed IUI, the first-line treatment for unexplained infertility, was the answer to our woes. IUI is basically sex 2.0, a technological upgrade on a primitive act. Conception hinges on the egg and the sperm meeting, but there is a very narrow window for that to occur, only two to six days in a menstrual cycle. IUI heightens the chances of the meeting taking place by picking up the best sperm from the male partner and depositing it in the uterus just as the egg emerges from the ovaries. The airlift not only ensures that the sperm reach on time, but also that at least a few hundred thousand of the most elite troopers are available at the site of action, having bypassed the long, perilous journey from the vagina to the uterus. IUI is thus sex better-timed and in the most optimal position.

'Sure, we can. If you don't want to give natural cycles a try, I understand. We can schedule an IUI next month.'

'Thanks,' I said, and turned to look at Ranjith. He remained blank, neutral to the discussion in the room. I was thrilled that we were going to implement a concrete course of action, but he was annoyingly impassive.

On the drive back home I tried to unscrew his tightly shut emotions.

'I really think IUI will work for us. It might take two or three attempts, but it will work. I have a strong gut feeling about this.'

'Hmm.'

'What do you think?'

He said nothing, his eyes not straying from the traffic.

'Why can't you say something? I need to know you are on board.'

'Yeah, I am OK with this, assuming the doctor knows what she is doing.'

'Yeah, but what do you think? Do you believe IUI will work? Do you think we are doing the right thing?'

'See, I don't know anything about this, and I don't want to know. I trust you and the doctor. I don't need to know all the details, it's immaterial.'

'Still, why can't you show some interest? Some involvement? You behave as if this has nothing to do with you. You don't even look like you are particularly interested in the outcome.'

'I don't know what you are talking about.'

'Ranjith?'

'Have you made lunch, or should we pick up something on the way?'

I sighed and backed off into my corner of resentful silence and incomprehension. If I pushed him any further, he would retreat into the black hole of his emotional universe. I was demanding more than he was ready to part with. He wanted to have a child; he had expressed that desire categorically. But he did not want to get down and dirty in the trenches of fertility medicine. Even consulting a doctor was a big step for him. Expecting a hands-on front-line approach from him was unrealistic. So, despite my best efforts to drag him into the centre-field, Ranjith remained a casual spectator, cheering occasionally from the stands. He entered the clinic, but his eyes never left sight of the exit.

3

What's a Lemon Squeezer Doing in My Vagina?

I heard of 'artificial insemination' for the first time in a Malayalam movie when I was eight or nine years old. It was Malayalam cinema's cult classic *Dasharatham* (1989), which was so ahead of its time that even now I am not sure if its time has come. A leading mainstream actor, Mohanlal, plays a rich, spoilt man-child who decides to act on a whim and have a child through surrogacy. He finds a desperate woman who needs money for her ailing footballer husband's medical treatment and agrees to rent her womb. They draw up a contract, turn up for the procedure, and fifteen days later she is pregnant! No failed attempts, cancelled cycles or any other complications. With this movie lodged in my brain for reference, I thought fertility treatments were an easy-peasy lemon-squeezy affair. To be fair to the movie, it is not about infertility. It's about a healthy, fertile couple who use artificial insemination for conception. It may well have happened that quickly and effortlessly in real life too. But the movie glosses over the unseemliness and hardships of the treatment. For those who have seen the movie, I hate to burst your bubble. Welcome to the world of ART.

I began our first IUI in July 2011 with the earnestness of a debutant, expecting early and prompt success. I had not dealt with sickness or physical incapacity in any significant manner until then, being blessed with a constitution that rarely fell prey to illness. I sailed through ten years of school without any noteworthy episodes of fever. My haemoglobin level typically hovered near the fourteen mark. When Ranjith caught the swine flu, despite my being in close contact with him my natural immunity provided the necessary shield against the deadly virus. My good health was my secret pride and I had taken it for granted all my life, expecting the body to tag along in whichever direction I pulled it. Therefore when we started treatment I anticipated the same level of responsiveness and performance from it. But for the first time, my body, specifically the reproductive apparatus, proved to be a terrible let-down, insolently ignoring my instructions.

The procedure itself was relatively simple with only a few key steps. The first step was pills to stimulate my ovaries to release multiple eggs. The second was follicular study. Follicles are tiny fluid-filled balloons in the ovaries that function as the home of the egg. They may expand from the size of a sesame seed (2 millimetres) to the size of a large kidney bean (18 mm to 25 mm) during the course of the menstrual cycle, eventually bursting to push the egg out. The follicles are measured at regular intervals during a cycle to ascertain if they have matured and are ready to release the egg. This is done through a transvaginal ultrasound (TVS).

I was not a big fan of TVS. It involved insertion of a long, slim plastic probe into my vagina and twisting it around to get a close look at the uterus. Magnified images of the uterus appeared on a computer screen. I was appalled the first time when the doctor covered the transducer with a condom and dipped it in lubricating gel, indicating that it had to enter an orifice in my body. I thought that scans, by definition, were non-invasive. It caused some discomfort, but it was not very painful. Eventually, I learnt to relax my muscles and spread my legs far apart to make things easier. I wished I didn't have to get a TVS, but if I had to then I could tolerate it.

The cycle got off on the wrong foot from the very beginning. The first ultrasound showed only one big-enough follicular blob (at 13 mm). The other four or five follicles were too small, indicating they might not reach maturity. This meant I might have only one egg despite taking drugs to stimulate the release of many.

In the next ultrasound, my ovarian plight did not show improvement. The lead follicle was still only at 15 mm (way below the 18 mm mark of maturity) and the others had not grown at all, looking like they were giving up on ovulation altogether.

There were no outward symptoms to show if the follicles were fattening or dying (this is true for most reproductive processes). So at every ultrasound I went in expecting miracle growth, only to be told that my seeds were lagging poorly behind. I felt helpless at the response from my body because there was nothing I could do to expand the follicles. If it were an outwardly manifest condition I could have applied my inner reserves of resolve and determination to improve the outcomes, in the same way that I would do daily exercise and physiotherapy to regain strength in an injured leg. But my action, or inaction, had no bearing on the ungovernable follicles.

We waited a couple of more days and did a third ultrasound. This time the news was worse. The lead follicle had ruptured; it hadn't waited for the others to catch up or even to reach its own full maturity. There was nothing left to do but to hurriedly put the sperm inside the uterus since an egg (presumably underdeveloped) had arrived and was waiting. The sperm transfer was scheduled for the same day.

I rang up my manager and said I would be taking the day off to address a personal emergency. An hour later, Ranjith drove in from his office to give a semen sample. He came in, gave the semen sample and left. He did not stay any longer because he had meetings that could not be rescheduled at such short notice.

I had come to the clinic at eight in the morning assuming I would just pop in for the ultrasound and pop out. An easy day with only the bother of TVS. But when I heard that I would have to stay back for the IUI, I inwardly experienced a mini-heart attack. Early on, while describing the procedure, Dr Leela had mentioned that the sperm would be *injected* inside the uterus using a *catheter*. Having heard the words 'inject' and 'catheter' in conjunction with my vagina, I thought it best to look up the process in detail on the Internet. One of the first search results showed that during an IUI the doctor uses a 'speculum' to pass the catheter into the uterus. It was a surgical instrument inserted inside the vagina or anus to dilate the area and give the doctor a better view. I did a quick search on Google Images to know what it looked like. The photos that flashed on my screen sent ripples of shock through my system. It looked like the stainless-steel *lemon squeezer* found in a kitchen. It was made of metal and about the same size as the kitchen tool. It had two blades to widen and hold open the vagina and a third handle with a screw to lock the instrument into place.

I clicked on multiple images, opened various websites, checking and cross-checking this. How could it be true? What would a lemon squeezer be doing in my vagina? Clearly, the vagina was not designed for anything this cold, sharp or hard. Besides, it is wide enough as it is for a plastic tube to pass through. Why wedge in an iron-and-steel contraption to keep it open? All kinds of reasoning raced up and down my non-medical brain, trying to discredit the barbaric speculum. Now that the IUI was only a few hours away I prayed that my information was wrong.

It was a busy day at the hospital for Dr Leela, who was swamped with several emergency C-sections. I sat alone in the deserted waiting hall of the IVF clinic, biding my time. Other patients had left after their ultrasounds in the morning. No one else was lined up for a procedure.

There were no magazines to read, no TV to watch in the white-tiled, white-walled, silver-chaired clinic. The nurses were huddled in the recovery room inside. The assistant doctor sat inside Dr Leela's cabin finishing paperwork. A lone receptionist kept me company. In an attempt at some conversation, I asked her redundantly if it was okay to drive myself back home after the IUI.

'Two-wheeler or four-wheeler?'

'Four-wheeler.'

'That's okay, then.'

Those were the only words we exchanged in the three hours spent in the same five hundred square feet of walled space.

When I got tired of sitting, I walked around the room, arms crossed over my chest. I stood at the glass windows, staring at the cars and people entering and exiting the parking lot below. Then I read and reread the IVF pamphlets on a magazine rack. The white, sterile silence was distressing; a sense of foreboding was closing in like a gathering storm. I struggled to banish the images of the lemon squeezer from my head.

Finally, at around one, Dr Leela came and apologized for the delay. I was taken to the operating room, asked to remove my leggings and empty my bladder. I lay down on the bed and pulled a sheet over my naked legs. A tray of surgical instrument kits was placed on a stand next to the bed. I kept my fingers crossed, hoping there would be no speculum.

Dr Leela began briskly tearing the kits open one by one and getting ready for action. When she pulled out the speculum, I lost my nerve. The thin mask of composure I was wearing until then crumbled. I sprang up and held back her hand desperately.

'Please, don't. I am scared.'

As soon as I said it, I regretted it. What was I thinking? It was a meaningless request. And Dr Leela had no patience for such trembling and dithering. She was not known to offer empty, placatory words, 'It's okay. Just relax. It will not hurt you.' My protest was an annoying interruption and she reacted sternly.

'Take your hand off. I don't need it here.'

The room became tense.

One of the nurses placed a finger on her lips and motioned me to be quiet and take deep breaths. They knew that upsetting the doctor was not in anybody's interest. I held the nurse's hand tightly, closed my eyes and willed myself to pull through this test. Dr Leela struggled to push the instrument in because my muscles were tight and wound-up.

'It is just not going in. You have to loosen up. This won't do,' she said, doubly frustrated.

The ninety seconds it must have taken to fix the speculum and inject the semen were excruciating, and not just because of the physical hostility of the act. Not just because it felt raw or sore or I was bleeding. But because it was a breach of my already fragile self. It tore through the membranes of my defences, leaving me exposed and helpless.

In a few minutes, it was over and the doctor left. The stainless-steel tools were taken out by the nurses. The housekeeping staff cleaned the floor. The room became empty again. The pounding in my heart ceased. I rested in the metallic stillness of the operating room for thirty minutes, drove home, ate my lunch and went to sleep.

That IUI was an eye-and-mind-opener of the path ahead. An IVF clinic is a cold place to walk into. It doesn't matter which IVF clinic you go to. There might be a difference in degree, but the air is still chilly and biting. You must shed your inhibitions, modesty and fears quickly because the most crucial part of fertility treatment involves lying on your back, knees bent, legs wide open, while probes, catheters and lemon squeezers are thrust inside your vagina by professionals whose day job this is. What you need is the stance of a warrior, not the long-suffering bearing of a patient.

~

Years later, I am just a few weeks away from going into labour. Ranjith's mother and I are alone at home. We are having a woman-to-woman conversation about the trials and tribulations of bringing a human into this world. We discuss pregnancy scans and the improvements in technology since her time. She speaks about her own repulsion and discomfort during an internal examination, which was necessary in her days when ultrasounds were not as prevalent.

She asks casually, only half-asking, but mostly reconfirming, 'You've never had an internal examination, *alle*?'

I gasp and mumble something to the effect of, 'Yes, I have.'

But the truth is, there was no short answer to that question.

4

Turning Point

Anyone who has been through school in India knows the hype surrounding class ten board exams. By the time you are in class eight, teachers, parents and neighbours will let you know that you are at a 'turning point' in your life. Everything from this juncture onwards is a build-up for the great climax. You are told that the class ten board exams are the summit, the last and the highest peak to conquer in the life of a school student. The exams have the power to propel you into the sphere of success, achievement and prosperity or to push you into the wretched hell-holes of failure and oblivion, sealing your fate for all eternity. This is where the winners and the losers get separated for the first time. This is where you are told, inarguably, what your place is in this world. Class ten exams are really do or die for Indians.

Like any self-respecting teen, I sneered at such spiel. Maybe the exams were a big deal if you wanted to opt for science or maths and enter an institution which excluded anyone below an aggregate score of 110 per cent. But I had no such ambition. I was a slightly better-than-average student and my sights were firmly fixed on the arts. I didn't have to succumb to this pressure. This was just another year, just another exam.

~

My father was a bank officer and my mother taught at the university. My brother (younger by two years) and I were born and raised in Trivandrum, where getting a good quality education was prized above all else. Even though there was constant bickering about money in the house, we went to the best convent schools in town. Amma never failed to remind us that education was the singular asset we had, and that the only means to come up through the ranks of society was a salaried job. Achan took great pride in recounting his own academic accomplishments, letting us know that we had a lot to live up to.

But most parents in Trivandrum then tended to have a limited definition of education. The two legitimate career choices before any student were engineering and medicine. The only reason you opted for arts or commerce was because you couldn't get an engineering or medicine seat on merit or your parents couldn't afford to buy one through the management quota. In which case you were met with thinly veiled contempt and pity. Your family's social prestige derived from the total of your marks scored in the tenth and twelfth standard board exams and your ranking in the common entrance exams for professional courses. For engineering students the icing on the cake was if you secured campus placement in TCS, Infosys or Satyam, at which point you had actualized your parents' dreams and fulfilled your life's purpose.

I believed in the benefits of a quality education, but I had no interest or aptitude for science and maths. English and history were my favourite subjects, neither of which even counted as 'worthwhile' subjects of study. By the time I was in class ten I had decided that I would choose a stream known as 'fifth group' for the two-year pre-degree course that followed. The different subject combinations for pre-degree education were called 'groups'. The first and second groups comprising science and maths were the most sought after. Next in the pecking order came 'fourth group', offering commerce. Those who didn't have the marks to be placed in any of these three had to be content with 'third group' or 'fifth group'. No one really *chose* 'third group' or 'fifth group'; they reconciled themselves to it. But even before I wrote my class ten finals I knew that I was going for 'fifth group' because it was a combination of all my favourite subjects—English literature, history and economics.

If I told someone that I was going to sign up for 'fifth group', their first response would be, 'What is that?' And then, 'Why? Can't you get into any other group?' If I explained that this was what I wanted to do, they would continue to look nonplussed. A small minority assumed that I was perhaps preparing to become an IAS officer. There is a third career option acceptable to parents in Trivandrum, and that is writing the Union Public Service Commission exam to become an officer in the Indian Foreign Service, Indian Administrative Service, Indian Police Service, or in any one of the twenty-odd categories of services that formed the Indian bureaucracy. So if you were a bright student and had still opted for 'third group' or 'fifth group', people concluded you were aiming for the esteemed civil services.

It was convenient to let them harbour this hope. *Why shatter other people's dreams for your future?*

Amma had set a modest goal for her two children: we had to be among the top ten in class. I would scrape through every time, getting the eighth or ninth rank. Once in a while I would make it to the top five, but that was rare. My strengths were English and social studies. Until class eight I could handle science and maths. But once in high school, there was a leap in the difficulty level of these subjects and I found myself floundering. I got into the pattern of only studying those subjects or chapters that I comprehended easily. This meant large swathes of physics, maths and even Hindi (which was my second language) dropped off my radar. My ranking in class also slipped—I was no longer among the top ten.

I was worried about my falling grades but I convinced myself that I could slog during the last three months before the exams and cover lost ground. But when I hit the last mile it became clear that making a late sprint to the victory post was not so simple. How was it possible to make up for years of sloth in one or two months? In subjects like physics and maths it was not possible to mug up textbooks. I had to understand theoretical concepts and apply them to solve problems, but my functional grasp of ideas was very weak. As a teenager I spent hours daydreaming about film stars and cricketers, scribbling in my diary, watching late-night TV shows and Test matches, and talking to classmates on the phone. I did not have the discipline or motivation to lock myself in my room and bury my head in the textbooks for hours on end.

Weeks of 'study holidays' passed, and the gap between my intentions and actions continued to widen while those around me prepared themselves for my academic baptism. Amma took fifteen days off from the university to be my chauffeur so that I did not have to wager on public bus services during the class ten boards. Achan's cousin who lived in Trivandrum visited us the day before the first exam solely to wish me luck. Grandparents, uncles and aunts, first and second cousins, all called to wish me. I felt guilty accepting each offer of best wishes, knowing that I was ill-prepared for the Olympic event.

I sat for the subject exams, one after the other, spread over three weeks, living up to my biases. I cruised through English, history and geography. The maths and science papers, on the other hand, were impenetrable. Entire sections were abandoned, I being unable to decode the mystic workings of graphs, formulas and equations. Amma, ever the pragmatist, had set a reasonable target. She said anything above an 80 per cent score was acceptable. I spent the entire summer break in prayer, hoping that by some fluke I could cross this barrier. I filled up notebooks speculating on the percentages I would score in each subject, adjusting the numbers again and again until I hit 80 per cent.

In the last week of May 1997, the ICSE Board announced the class ten results. The Internet was still two years away from reaching our homes so we had to go to the school to check the scores. When I entered the arches of the brick building the mood was one of jubilation and victory. The school had recorded one of its best performances until then. Student after student ran through the results in the sheet pinned on the glass-cased notice board and the grins got wider. Teachers were seen congratulating students and parents thanking the teachers in tearful gratitude. Amma and I walked into this atmosphere of celebration, our hearts quaking and trembling with anxiety.

We met one of my classmates who was hopping down the staircase, on her way out. She was ecstatic because she had scored 85 per cent. Sensing my nervousness, she said encouragingly, 'Everyone has done very well. Even those who scored 60 per cent in the pre-boards have scored above 80 per cent. So you have nothing to worry about.' My spirits lifted. I pushed my way through the crowd of girls jostling near the notice board to find my name on the list. Yes, everyone had done exceedingly well. Even those who were not expected to. Most students had scored above 80 per cent. And I had scored 78.6 per cent.

I went back to Amma, hid my face in her chest and sobbed uncontrollably, muttering my score in between tears. One or two friends came by to inquire. I didn't lift my face from the folds of her by-now-wet saree. The grief and shame sat so heavily on my shoulders. What made it worse was that I was the outlier; there was no one else to share my failure.

Amma said, 'It's OK, *mole*,' and rubbed my back, but her disappointment was no less than mine. When her colleagues called to inquire about her daughter's score, she avoided mentioning the precise number. She indicated it was nothing to write home about.

Obviously, scoring an aggregate of 78.6 per cent did not warrant such a breakdown. It was certainly not the apocalyptic disaster that I made it out to be. But I had just missed the 80 per cent mark. In our universe then, 80 per cent meant distinction, it meant respectability, it meant crossing the threshold of success . . . and I had faltered just short of it.

Before the results came out, Amma was nudging me towards taking up science for my pre-degree course. She suggested that I could always do arts for graduation but if I gave up science and maths at this stage there was no going back to it later. But once the marks were out she stopped these arguments. With this aggregate it was difficult to secure admission into the science stream of any of the better-known schools or colleges. I could always get a seat in the same school where I had studied so far, but I didn't fancy going back there. I had lost face by howling in front of all my classmates—how could I look them in the eye again? My marks sheet showed that I scored the highest marks in English and the lowest in physics. There was no hiding the fact that my strength lay in the arts. Achan also reminded Amma that forcing me to labour through another two years of science was like insisting that fish climb trees (from the famous Einstein analogy).

So I applied to one of the few private colleges in the city which offered the 'fifth group'. A friend's mother taught here. She assured Amma that I could get admission because 'fifth group' didn't have many takers. And if I didn't she would put in a word for me. When the college put out the merit list of selected students, mine was the last name. It was a choice I would have made anyway, but now it was the only choice left to make. And I didn't like that feeling.

I was separated from my friends who opted to carry on in the same school. In college the brightest students gravitated towards science or commerce, and the pool of students left to do 'third group' or 'fifth group' were in some sense the 'castaways', except for a few. It had neither the prestige and approval of 'first group' and 'second group', nor the glamour and swagger of 'fourth group'. If you said 'fifth group', you automatically nose-dived to the bottom of the college popularity index. My pride, by now, was dead and cremated; only ash and wisps of smoke remained. Well, what do you know! Class ten boards *are* a turning point. *Why hadn't anyone told me that?*

Almost overnight, the composition of my personality changed. It was now laced with feelings of shame and underachievement. I had let down my parents and surely didn't deserve the facilities they had provided me. Instead of repaying their trust I had defrauded them of their life's investments. I felt I didn't deserve to be valued or respected or cared for until I undid the damage. I came to believe that the sum total of my worth rested on what marks I could score in a particular examination, on my numerical position in relation to a measurable goal. This gave birth to my lifelong obsession with numbers, with performance, with success. So when I confronted infertility and seemed to be tumbling down loops of failure, the same feelings of shame and disgrace welled up inside. It lacerated my thirty-year-old self-esteem in exactly the same manner my class ten score had affected my fifteen-year-old one.

5

If Ever an IUI Was Destined to Work, This Was It

It was a six-hour overnight flight back from Istanbul, where we had gone on our first foreign holiday. I sat cross-legged on the economy seat, wrapped in a blanket, and watched three Hollywood romcoms back to back, foregoing sleep completely. A few hours earlier we had been walking the labyrinthine lanes of Grand Bazaar when a headache started. At first a dull ache, later a metronomic throb. It was fifteen days after the sperm transfer, around the time at which I was due to find out if the first IUI had worked. Inferring this headache to be a sure-shot sign of pregnancy, we walked to the nearest pharmacy and bought a home pregnancy test. I decided to use it the next morning, once we landed in India.

The doctor had not explicitly banned travel. We didn't cross-check with her either before planning the overseas trip. I thought the six-day holiday to Turkey would be a welcome distraction from the twenty-four-hour 'Am I pregnant?' self-interrogation underway. On the holiday there was time

to ask that question only a few times every day, mostly as
an afterthought before going to sleep. But there was also a
nagging worry as to whether I was exceeding my quota of
blessings—a foreign holiday and a pregnancy in the same
fortnight? Could I have both?

It was four in the morning when we landed in Bangalore.
The tarmac was awash in the harsh white of the floodlights.
My eyes were burning from a sleepless night as we stepped off
the airport bus at the international terminal. I walked briskly
to the restroom, while Ranjith stood outside guarding our
backpacks. I chose the first stall that was empty, fished out
the test from my handbag and scanned the instructions on
the leaflet. After dropping my urine in the test well, I waited,
utterly still, except for the thud-thud of my heart. A short
streak of red appeared. I continued to wait. Just the single
line. I counted to fifty, slowly, deliberately. Still nothing. Just
the short streak of red. A sigh escaped my chest and I flung
the test in the dustbin and walked out, not looking back or
slowing down. I went to Ranjith who was waiting outside; he
didn't have to ask, and I didn't have to tell. This trip was over.

~

The failure of the first IUI was disappointing. When the
cramping and bleeding of my period started, I spent the first
day crying my usual tears. Yet it did not bring our lives to a
grinding halt. This was our first attempt, and from my Internet
sources I knew that the first IUIs, IVFs, rarely work. More
critically, we did not have a show-stopping cycle, only one
lead follicle, and that too had burst hastily, releasing a half-
baked egg. I was also going through a phase of tremendous

pressure at work, having been given the responsibility of leading a ten-member team for the first time. Caught between a new, important and demanding client on the one hand and aggrieved and overworked colleagues on the other, my career as a professional juggler was in full flight. There were client demos, hiring interviews, new-joiner trainings, escalations, performance feedback sessions and hundreds of emails that swarmed into my inbox every hour to colonize all my attention. I was logged into the computer from six in the morning till eleven in the night, but my mind was running twenty-four hours of the day, seven days of the week. Stress was piling up by the day and I calculated that it must have played a silent role in killing my baby hopes.

And the work itself? Well, knowledge management seemed like a performance staged in front of a near-empty hall. Most of it involved maintaining a large internal website or a 'knowledge portal' for the use of employees within the organization. I belonged to the team that managed and maintained this website. Our work included creating web pages, uploading documents, and sending out communications alerting employees about the pages created and documents uploaded. The content on the portal was meant to capture internal best practices and facilitate collaboration among peers. But I suspected that few employees accessed it of their own volition; they had to be compelled by appraisal requirements. The only people who voluntarily used the portal were the ones who created and maintained it. That's us. It was a self-perpetuating exercise, our work primarily meant to justify our own existence.

From an 'analyst', I grew to be a 'senior analyst' and then a 'specialist'. But the work remained the same. At social gatherings, I would panic if someone asked me what I did for a living. On those occasions I envied my brother; he could fling a single, all-encompassing word—'software'—and walk away in slow motion to approving nods from everyone in the room. That word communicated not just his line of work but his educational background, professional goals, financial standing, social status, political views, retirement plans . . . his entire human existence was encapsulated in those two syllables. I, on the other hand, had to summon up a plethora of jargon and spout them in random combinations, 'Tacit knowledge, explicit knowledge, knowledge harvesting, knowledge transfer, knowledge this, knowledge that . . .' to little effect.

I longed to have a career which centred on 'real-world' problems, such as curing an ailment, constructing a building, educating a child or writing a book, which could be easily understood and explained. And which had a direct connection with the world outside, and a beneficial impact on society. The purpose of knowledge management was so obscure and the skills that it needed were so generic! On most days all my role needed was a high school education and, possibly, attention to detail.

Each day, I sat at my laptop in the morning, reviewed fresh tasks from our internal clients in the US and deftly assigned them to my team. The tasks were logged in an online tracking system, and the metrics it generated were viewed with utmost seriousness. We hailed employees for addressing the largest number of client requests. A five-star rating on a request was applauded. Reward points were doled out for exceptional work. But what did it all amount to? How many lives did we save? Or what did we develop? Or what did we make more efficient or effective? The work, I felt, had little relevance outside the office floor the team occupied. Entering that building was like arriving in a parallel universe, successfully isolated from worldly concerns. All the work that I did began in my mail inbox and ended in the client's inbox, safely hidden from all humanity, only fished out while filling out self-assessment sheets.

Since the day I joined the company I had been considering quitting, but I kept postponing the decision. The next thing I knew, I had spent five years in knowledge management and become a 'domain expert'. But the work was not inspiring, and the higher I grew in the organization the more difficult it became to maintain the myth of work-life balance. The office space demanded 24x7 involvement from an individual who had nothing else to do and no one else to deal with. For me, this life was untenable. Therefore I wondered if should continue doing work that didn't galvanize my heart or brain and at the same time swallowed up all my waking hours. Was it worthwhile? And what were my life goals? If I wanted to have a baby and if that meant ART, then this lifestyle was hardly helping. We had to commit ourselves exclusively to the demands of the treatment; half-hearted attempts were hurting our chances.

This was the reasoning in my mind as I persuaded myself, and in the process Ranjith too, into believing that the *job* was the hurdle that lay between us and the baby. It was therefore my moral obligation to eliminate it before restarting infertility treatment. I chose a Friday evening and ambushed my manager with the resignation email, writing about my own disillusionment with the job and corporate life. I also made it clear that for now I was going to take a break from working itself to focus on some domestic priorities. My manager was kind enough to offer a variety of flexible working arrangements to accommodate my personal interests, but my mind was set on giving up my job altogether. I believed it had to be one or the other. No middle ground was possible. On 19 October 2011, soon after our first failed IUI, I surrendered my laptop and access card and left the building, proud and fully confident that I was choosing a new direction in life and bringing Ranjith and me closer to having a baby.

~

Two days later I flew to Trivandrum to help Amma with my brother's impending wedding. The first few days of unemployment felt like walking out of confinement, and I spent the next three weeks finding joy in being Amma's chief assistant wedding planner. Once the celebrations were over, it was back to Bangalore to begin our second IUI. In December 2011, we went back to the same clinic, this time bringing single-minded focus and determination to the examination table.

Dr Leela increased the dosage of the ovulation stimulating medication, given the poor response it fetched in the previous attempt. Thankfully, my ovaries rose to the challenge and by day twelve of the menstrual cycle there were four plump, ripe follicles brimming with eggs inside. The uterine lining thickened adequately in preparation for fertilization. A shot of the hCG hormone was given to complete the maturation of the follicles and trigger the release of eggs. About forty hours after the hCG shot, the sperm transfer would be done.

It was a Saturday. We went to the clinic in the morning for an ultrasound to check if the follicles had burst. I was experiencing sharp ovulation pain on the right side of my abdomen, deceptively similar to menstrual aches. I assumed that the follicles had burst and the eggs were floating around waiting for their sperm beaus. But the ultrasound threw a surprise; the follicles had not ruptured yet. If in the last IUI my egg came too early, this time it was late to the party.

'Let's wait for some more time. We can do another ultrasound in the afternoon and then do the IUI after the follicles have ruptured. That way the timing will be perfect,' Dr Leela suggested.

Ranjith and I went home and waited. At one in the afternoon we came back to the hospital. The second ultrasound had to be done in the main hospital facility because the radiologist was available in the IVF clinic only for a few hours in the morning. By now the scan showed that the lead follicle, a voluptuous 22 mm, had split wide open. We took the report to the IVF clinic, but Dr Leela was not available. So we continued to wait.

As with the first IUI, this time too there was a lot of waiting. The waiting exacerbated my anxiety. My hands and toes were cold and clammy, and my stomach rumbled and churned all day. I didn't eat anything after breakfast. Having Ranjith around was comforting to some extent; I had someone to talk to and lean on. But it didn't do much good for my jumpy nerves because what I was most worried about I had to face alone—the lemon squeezer.

IUI is now offered under general anaesthesia in some clinics. I would have gratefully paid the extra fees for being knocked out if the option had been available then, but there were no such alternatives. We spent all afternoon waiting for Dr Leela in uneasy silence. I did not want to go home or even to the cafeteria in the main hospital—what if we missed her?

At four, Sini, the Malayalee nurse, came out to the waiting area and motioned me inside. They had word from Dr Leela to prepare the patient; she would be in the clinic in half an hour. I undressed, put on the hospital gown and emptied my bladder. Sini brought a steel lab tray to my bed. There was an injection prior to the IUI. This was new.

'This is to help the uterus relax,' she explained.

Grateful for the tranquillizing medicine, I lay on my side while she pricked my buttocks, forcing the 'relaxing' liquid into my bloodstream. Like I said earlier, I am not scared of needles or cannulas, but that jab caused such a stinging, reverberating pain that I let out a cry in shock.

'What was that?'

'It's an oil-based injection. They tend to be more painful.'

'Tell me about it.'

I got up and rubbed the spot vigorously with my hands, trying to soothe the sore skin and muscle.

'Ithinekallum bhedam speculum aanallo,' I told Sini. I preferred the speculum to this shot.

She smiled a knowing smile.

Soon, Dr Leela arrived and I went into the IUI room. By now the lemon squeezer was at the top of my mind, but I had come prepared to stand up to my fears. Not all women found it as gut wrenching as I did. The more relaxed I was the easier it would be for me and the doctor. Besides, I could not wish it away, and the only reasonable response was to take the speculum head-on. I started repeating some affirmations and motivational phrases looked up the day before in my head:

'I am strong, brave and open to this experience.'

'My body can take this easily and effortlessly.'

'No pain, no gain.'

I locked my hands over my chest, folded my legs and closed my eyes, cutting myself off from the action in the room, silently reciting the phrases. There was the rustle and crackle of kits opening, the clinking and clanking of metal. Dr Leela spewed terse instructions to her crew.

In a few seconds the cold mass of stainless steel entered and I felt chafing inside as Dr Leela tightened the screws. But I kept my calm, concentrating on taking loud, deep breaths.

Dr Leela acted quickly, sliding the plastic catheter in without an iota of hesitation to slow down her rhythm. Someone brought the semen sample and it was injected inside. I kept my eyes closed and my breathing forceful, thinking all along, 'When is the damn thing coming out?'

In a few minutes it was over. The speculum was unscrewed and withdrawn. My muscles relaxed. I lowered my legs. My breathing eased up, even and involuntary again.

'All the best. Let's hope it works this time,' Dr Leela said, before leaving the room.

I rested on the bed, quietly proud of having held myself together, all in one piece.

I faced the speculum many, many times after this with descending levels of fear and paranoia and ascending degrees of calmness and composure. It stopped being the central horror to confront and overcome in my infertility journey. It fell from its top-ranking position and jostled for space with the TVS, injections and pills—an unpleasantness, like a prickly cactus whose thorns brush against your skin causing discomfort but no injury. A small mound of courage slowly accumulated in place of the disarray and helplessness. I told myself each time that if I can do this once, I can do it again. Yet, every time the speculum was wedged inside, time stood still. For the two or three minutes I had to last with a steel apparatus sticking out from my vagina, my body snapped to a state of extreme attentiveness while my mind tried to zone out, dissociate itself from the physical event. It never became fully easy, just progressively less difficult.

The IUI took place on 17 December 2011. The beta hCG blood test to detect a pregnancy is usually ordered exactly fifteen days after the IUI. This would have meant 31 December 2011, which was a Saturday. Dr Leela postponed it to 2 January 2012 for a more propitious timing, believing the New Year would reverse my fertility fortunes. While leaving the clinic I clasped Sini's hands—she had seen me through the procedure—and said, 'Please pray for me.' She responded unhesitatingly with 'Sure, definitely.' I was happy that someone unrelated to me had agreed to say prayers for my sake; the combined pleas must align astrological forces and result in a pregnancy, I thought.

In my estimation we had ticked all the boxes. Our lives were adequately primed to receive a baby. Job eliminated. Stress zero. Even the obligatory first failure was out of the way. The follicles had developed to their full potential. The transfer of sperm to the uterus had progressed comfortably with none of the drama of the previous attempt. This was a best-case IUI, an IUI maximum. An IUI born from the perfect intersection of science, body and faith. If ever an IUI was destined to work, *this* was it.

Dr Leela had not prescribed any special care or precaution during the waiting period, no restrictions against travelling or strenuous activity. So Ranjith and I decided to spend the last week of the year driving out of town to Ottappalam in Kerala. Ranjith's parents lived here, having bought a house in the small town after retirement to be close to their siblings.

Ottappalam was a charming dot on Kerala's map with green hills, coconut trees and paddy fields sprawled all over its landscape. The town centre comprised a narrow, sinuous road with rows of shops on either side, one 'family dining' restaurant and a few single-screen cinema halls. Here, 'party' meant Congress or CPI-M, and New Year's Eve meant nothing. I felt a little blue turning our backs on the seductions of the holiday season and driving into the blankness of a town untouched by urban frills. But Ranjith, in sharp contrast, embraced the setting wholeheartedly. He assimilated into that milieu instantly, tucking in his mundu and tuning in to talk on the week's rainfall, temple festivals and family gossip.

On New Year's Eve we obediently followed Ranjith's parents to all the obligatory temples and homes of uncles and aunts, ate dinner at eight, watched TV till nine and retired to bed by nine-thirty. Ranjith, happy and content with a day well-spent, began to snore as soon as he hit the pillow, while I remained bright and awake, twiddling my thumbs on a phone that had no network, dreaming of all the places we could have been in. Soon, I too made peace with the inertia and fell asleep, short-term pleasures written off for long-term goals.

The next day we drove back to Bangalore and to urban civilization. When we were about to enter RR Road, four kilometres from our house, a long line of traffic pile-up stopped us. Every car owner in Bangalore was heading back to the city after a vacation. We got pinned to the road for close to two hours, looking wistfully at our apartment complex that was almost in sight. I killed time in the car ringing up friends and family to wish them a Happy New Year but feeling none of the mirth projected in my voice. Both of us believed that the first day of a New Year is a portend of things to come, and this day had been botched up, not by some extraordinary event but by the most quotidian phenomenon of our cities. We were exhausted from the journey, frustrated with the delay and had to let go of our plans to eat out. It seemed a grim start to the New Year.

~

I began the two-week wait period for the pregnancy test in a rainbow-coloured bubble, buoyed up by fantasies of imminent motherhood. Somewhere deep within, I felt very keenly that it was bound to work this time. We had made all the necessary adjustments. The principles of natural justice dictated that this IUI result in a pregnancy. It was only fair! But as the days slipped past, one by one, the bubble shrank and burst, leaving behind only a soapy uncertainty. There was not a single physical sign of pregnancy that I could attest to despite all attempts at mentally manufacturing them. I googled every day for stories of women who did not have any symptoms and still got a positive pregnancy test. But the absence of any physical signs bore heavily on my mind. If I was pregnant, surely I would feel something, a twinge, a bulge, some wooziness, something different from my non-pregnant state? But I remained the same old infertile me.

By 2 January 2012, when I was scheduled to take the beta hCG test, my suspicions had hardened to a firm belief that this cycle too had failed. I drove myself to the clinic feeling downcast, while Ranjith left for office. Sini drew my blood sample for the test and wished me luck.

'I don't feel very confident,' I said.

'Why?'

'I don't have any symptoms.'

'Hmm.'

Her reticence only worsened my doubts. Three hours later, back at home, the call came. I immediately dialled Ranjith and my mother to give them the news, disconnecting the calls as soon as I had conveyed the result. Then I fell on my bed in a heap, like a tree felled to the ground. A slow and deep wail was rising from the centre of my being; a wail advancing like an all-conquering army, snuffing out each post of resistance in the way. I surrendered to the force of that wail.

A grim start to the New Year, indeed.

6

Time for the Big Guns

After the second IUI, I went through two more. But I went about these with a perfunctoriness that came from anger and dejection. Like a sulking child, I went through the motions resignedly, not with purpose or intention. I didn't even take time off to regroup. Between December 2011 and February 2012 I had three back-to-back IUIs—all drawing blanks. My uterus did put up a good show each time, producing four to five ripe follicles and a thickened endometrium, but inside I harboured no conviction that it would work—because if the second IUI which had my maximum investment had not brought the desired result, how was anything less going to suffice?

I also went through a hysteroscopy, which is believed to be the gold standard in the evaluation of infertility. The doctor inserts a tube with a light and camera into your vagina to take a deep look at the uterus for any irregularities. Mercifully, this procedure is done under anaesthesia. After the test Dr Leela proudly handed over a CD with the images of my uterus captured during the hysteroscopy. Everything was perfect.

There was nothing wrong in Ranjith's semen analysis either. She was pleased with her footage and exhorted us to view the images. 'What was the point?' we thought. If everything was so splendid why was I not getting pregnant? We still didn't have a medical reason to explain our inability to conceive.

Unexplained infertility is a conundrum—on the one hand, your reproductive system is deemed medically fit and fine. On the other, it is unable to perform the very function it was created for. After every round of investigations I felt disappointed to know that there was nothing significantly wrong, nothing which needed to be corrected. This meant going back to the roulette table and placing our bets on a random number. The odds were pretty much the same. If there was a fixable problem, it would have given us something concrete and tangible to work on and work towards, but instead we were shooting in the dark.

'The success rate of an IUI cycle is only 15 to 20 per cent, and most IUI pregnancies occur in the first three or four attempts,' Dr Leela said, practically. We were meeting her after the fourth failed IUI.

To me the IUI appeared to be only slightly better than sex—the sperm and egg still had to meet and fertilize on their own. The only advantage it offered was the timing and creation of proximity for the two to meet. It was increasingly looking like a waste of time and money. We needed something more robust and adaptive to coax my reproductive system to deliver.

'What about IVF?' I inquired.

'Yes, we can try that. But you don't have any serious problems which warrant it. Such as tubal damage, abnormal sperm or diminished ovarian reserve. And you are still quite young.'

'I know. But we have been married for six years and I don't want to wait any longer.'

I was thirty-one and Ranjith was thirty-five. We felt there was no point in squandering our precious reproductive years trying out procedures that had a limited success ratio. So we waited for four or five months after the last IUI and went back to Dr Leela asking for IVF.

Here the reader might get the impression that it was an easy and uncomplicated decision to make.

Scene One:

Ranjith and I sit across the table.

Ranjith: IUIs have failed. What should we do?

Me: IVF, of course.

Ranjith: Great! Let's do it then.

End of scene.

No, the conversation didn't quite pan out like that.

Emotionally and mentally, IUI was an easy call to make because it was quite close to natural conception. Dr Leela recommended that we have intercourse on the day of the IUI. So, if a cycle worked it left enough elbow room for us to believe that it may have happened 'naturally'. But IVF gave us no chance at feigning that it was 'natural'. Every stage of conception was controlled and manipulated, and fertilization was expected to take place in a laboratory, outside my uterus.

There were other reasons too stacked against IVF. It was exorbitantly expensive, a single IVF cycle potentially running up a bill upwards of one lakh fifty thousand rupees. To make matters worse, a single cycle would not be enough. We had to commit ourselves to at least three cycles to have a reasonable chance of success. The success rate for an IVF cycle in a good clinic is 30 per cent to 35 per cent. So, unless we signed up for three attempts, we were going into battle with too few cannonballs.

IVF was also a staggering commitment in terms of time and effort. It was IUI raised to the power of ten. I would have to make daily visits to the hospital for a month. During the first stage, known as ovarian hyperstimulation, drugs are injected into the woman's body to persuade the ovarian follicles to yield more eggs. Blood tests and ultrasounds are done every two to three days to assess how the reproductive system is faring. When the follicles have bloated up, the 'trigger shot' of hCG is given for final maturation of the eggs. Up until this point the process is similar to IUI, except that IVF is a higher-voltage version. But instead of just injecting the sperm inside the woman's body at this point, as in IUI, in IVF the doctor opts to wade in and retrieve the egg from the follicle because she doesn't trust the two to do the job on their own. Once the egg is picked up from the body it is handed over to an embryologist.

A few thousand sperm and the retrieved eggs are sent on a blind date by the embryologist, who just places them in a petri dish where they have the opportunity to hook up. For better results sometimes, a more aggressive procedure known as intra-cytoplasmic sperm injection (ICSI) is performed. The embryologist picks up a single sperm with a fine needle and pierces the egg with it, in an act of forced mating. If the sperm succeeds in fusing with the egg, an embryo results. An embryo is a single-cell entity, the grain-equivalent of a fully grown human being comprising trillions of cells. This microscopic life form is placed in an incubator for the next five to six days. It is expected to cleave symmetrically into two cells, then four, then eight and so on with each passing day.

On the third or fifth day after the egg retrieval procedure the embryo is typically transferred back into the woman's uterus where it must attach itself to the uterine lining to result in a pregnancy. Did I say there's nothing 'natural' about IVF?

I wanted IVF and I did not want IVF.

~

I had just returned to work after the break. When I quit my job I had subconsciously believed that excessive devotion to my career was the reason we didn't have a baby yet. Like so many women who have been told this all their lives, I too believed I couldn't have it all. So I 'sacrificed' my job at the altar of potential motherhood, making a votive offering and expecting immediate gains in return. I folded up my professional ambitions and placed them at destiny's feet saying, 'Here, take it. Now give me a baby.' There were right-minded reasons to let go of the job, independent of ART and pregnancy, but the primary motivation and the immediate trigger had been this. By the end of that year, when I had no job and no baby, it felt incredibly foolish. No, there was no exchange offer on careers and children. It occurred to me that a child had to fit into the existing segments of our lives; we could rearrange things a bit, but we could not empty out all the contents to make place for a baby. So after the failed IUIs I updated my resumé and started putting the word out. I sought a role in the development sector, which I presumed would be more fulfilling and meaningful than corporate life.

Before long I found a position in an NGO that worked on strengthening the school education system. There was some scope for applying my knowledge management skills from the earlier job, but mostly it was brand-new territory for me. From the structured, process-driven and deadline-directed world of corporations, I was entering the amorphous territory of social change. There was extensive reading to do on educational theory, philosophy, research and policy. I knew nothing about the RTE Act beyond its expanded form—the Right of Children to Free and Compulsory Education Act. I thought Khan Academy was another one of Salman Khan's philanthropic ventures. During the interview I claimed to know Kannada but failed to mention that my Kannada vocabulary was limited to four words: 'gudisi' (sweep), 'oresi' (mop), 'pathre' (vessels) and 'batte' (clothes). There was a lot of ground to cover at the level of discourse as well as ways of working. And in the middle of all this IVF was looking like a terrible nuisance.

An IVF cycle meant time off and flexible working hours. I would have to drive myself to the hospital every day, take my shots and then bounce back to work. The new office was fifteen kilometres away, and I was likely to be late by an hour or two for the first ten to twelve days of the cycle. Then I would need leave on the day of egg retrieval and embryo transfer. Perhaps a few more days off after the embryo transfer for rest. How could I negotiate this in a new job?

Moreover, even if we could work out the physical pressures and financial costs, I did not believe I could bear the psychological and emotional toll IVF entailed. It meant reopening old wounds and walking the same path that had only led us up a blind alley earlier. Between my IUI and IVF treatments, I found myself sane for the most part. I was content with my pleasant middle-class life revolving around job, husband and home. Once fertility treatment started, the lights would go out like the flick of a switch inside my brain, and gloom would descend. My full-scale life was now contracted to a single pinpoint. The IUI days began with the visit to the clinic; syringes and ultrasounds would follow. I obsessed over each step—the growth of my follicles, the thickness of my endometrium, my estradiol levels, my progesterone levels . . . no detail was too minute to not lose sleep over. Coupled with this everyday anxiety was the overarching anxiety about the outcome of the treatment. Will this work? Will I get pregnant this time? It was a fast-track path to insanity invented by humankind. An act of self-flagellation, really.

And there was no guarantee of success. Having experienced four failed IUIs in rapid succession, I no longer even believed that ART was destined to give us a baby. This is what repeated failure does to you; you stop believing in success. The heat to experience pregnancy and motherhood had cooled off because of the recurrent setbacks. In my heart, getting pregnant and having a child was a mirage. We could keep chasing it with whatever resources we were fortunate to have, but it remained a mirage. The further we walked, the more distant it seemed.

I agonized over the IVF decision for several months, shuttling back and forth, discussing it with Ranjith, my mother and my best friend from college, Sara. But I was only buying time, trying to defer a difficult call. Eventually, I came around and voted in favour of IVF. The biggest deciding factor was Ranjith himself. Ranjith's frame of mind had gone through a 180-degree shift. He had switched from believing that 'nothing is wrong' and therefore 'nothing needs to be done' to a battle-ready 'let's-throw-everything-we-have-plus-the-kitchen-sink-at-this' mode.

'We have to give IVF a try. Imagine being sixty and thinking if only we had done IVF.'

'It's easy for you to say. But I am the one who has to enter that hole. And what if even this doesn't work?'

'I know. If it doesn't work, it doesn't work. We are still at baseline. But at least we will have the satisfaction of knowing that we have done everything in our hands.'

Sometime in between, seeing my resistance to IVF, we contemplated the idea of adoption. We went to a child-care centre in Bangalore to talk to the authorities about the availability, waiting period and the paperwork involved. But we both recognized it was not for us. I didn't trust myself. Could I own a child not born to us? Would I do justice to her? Besides, a big part of wanting a child was the yearning to experience pregnancy and childbirth. I was not ready to forfeit that just yet.

So it all came down to this: Ranjith asked if I could and I said yes, not having the heart to say no. I submitted to his wishes because my own judgement was foggy. Age is a pivotal factor in reproductive medicine, especially maternal age. If, five years later, I changed my mind, I would be close to forty and my chances of success would have declined significantly. We had a limited time frame to fiddle with the dials and knobs of fertility medicine and I did not want to set myself up for regret later.

In the depths of my heart I also believed that IVF gave us our best shot at success. IVF meant that we could break down the process of conception stage by stage, step by step, and arm-twist it to achieve the outcomes we coveted. So, ultimately, over an SMS conversation with Ranjith in the middle of a working day, I took a deep breath and typed, 'Okay. Let's bring out the big guns.'

7

A Sperm and an Egg Are Not Equal

The first IVF cycle began in September 2012, about seven months after the last IUI had failed. Like the first IUI, this too was a certified disaster. My ovaries responded poorly to the medicine, producing only a few eggs and of dubious quality. Needless to say, no baby was born out of that cycle. But this was anticipated because the first cycle is used as a baseline to understand how the body works. IVF is like watching a food show on TV and then trying to recreate the dish at home by following the recipe. Even if you have the exact ingredients and measurements and follow the same techniques, the final product may not match the original inspiration. It takes repetition and practice. As with cooking, in IVF too there is a lot of trial and error. So the first cycle is a warm-up cycle, which gives the doctor insight into the problem areas— such as perhaps the number of eggs produced, egg quality, fertilization, embryo quality, thickness of the endometrium or implantation. It helps her dismantle the machinery of conception and peer at each constituent through a microscope to nail down what is not working optimally. The know-how gathered from the first cycle is then used to modulate various aspects of the treatment in the subsequent cycles.

After the sub-par response from my ovaries in the first IVF cycle, Dr Leela suggested that we try DHEA (dehydroepiandrosterone) tablets, a hormone used to treat women with shrinking ovarian reserves. Some research has shown that DHEA supplementation helps women improve their egg quality. I swallowed the DHEA pill every night for three months before starting the next cycle of treatment.

Dr Leela also ordered the anti-müllerian hormone (AMH) test. AMH is a hormone that indicates a woman's ovarian reserve. The higher the number of eggs left in the ovaries, the higher the level of AMH and the better the chances of conceiving. I had last tested AMH in 2011. It was 3.4 then; the reference range in the lab report being 2.0–6.38. Even then my AMH level was towards the lower end of the spectrum, but I was comfortably placed within the margins of what was considered 'normal'. Dr Leela wanted to review key ovarian statistics before starting the second cycle, because the egg was key to unlocking the fertility door.

Every woman is born with a finite number of eggs, which is on average a couple of millions. But this corpus of eggs continues to deplete in both count and quality with every passing year until it is completely empty. By the time a girl hits puberty, more than half her ovarian reserve may have vanished. There is no way to add more eggs to the basket. Every month during ovulation, follicles release one or more of the already-existing eggs. The quality of the egg released is strongly correlated with successful implantation and live birth. But the older the egg, the more likely it is to have chromosomal abnormalities. So there is only a limited number of eggs in the first place, and they dwindle in number and grade every year.

In contrast, each time an adult man ejaculates he may release 40 million to 1.2 billion sperm cells! This sperm army travels from the vagina to the fallopian tubes to meet the waiting egg. But this is a difficult journey, and all but one (if at all even one) will perish during its course. This explains why it takes millions of sperm to fertilize a single egg. Sperm cells have a longer life span than eggs (eggs only survive for twenty-four hours after ovulation) and can live for about four to five days inside the woman's body. While women stop ovulating after an age, men continue to produce sperm throughout their lives. While their sperm count and motility might reduce over the years, men remain capable of fathering a child well into their advanced years.

Therefore, the statement, 'you need one sperm and one egg to produce a baby', while being technically correct, creates a false equivalence between the two. In IVF terms, an egg is a far more prized commodity than a sperm. Getting one good-quality sperm cell is relatively easy—you have millions to pick from—while the stock of eggs is a hastily diminishing resource. This is why fertility treatment is mostly centred on the woman and her eggs. Even after the egg is retrieved and fertilized in a lab, the remaining work of reproduction is borne by the woman. Implantation, pregnancy, labour—everything happens inside the woman's body. And therefore it is the woman's body that is the site for all fertility interventions. Even in cases of male infertility, once the sperm has been retrieved from the man or donor sperm are employed, it's the woman who bears the brunt of the procedures. Infertility is *not* an equal-opportunity employer.

This inherent biological 'inequality' caused structural imbalances in our marriage. In our case, neither of us had any major issues, yet I was the one who was being treated. For the IUIs, I went alone for the shots, ultrasounds and blood work. For the first IVF, Ranjith accompanied me on the day of egg retrieval, because I had to be under general anaesthesia, and also on the day of the embryo transfer when his semen sample was required. On my other visits he had nothing to do. Even on the days he came along with me he was just sitting idly in the waiting area, staring at his phone. He didn't have to take an injection, pop a pill or undergo a surgical procedure. Perhaps this made him feel slightly irrelevant in the ART scheme of things. However, the goal of the treatment was for us to have a baby; it was a joint undertaking. But, given the manner in which fertility treatment panned out, his role turned out to be a side show.

Ranjith had no interest in the science of infertility. He did not read up on the topic. Even in the matter of decisions such as which doctor or clinic we should go to, he left them entirely to my judgement. He did not have any questions for the doctor; he was a silent accomplice. He assumed that she was doing her best and that we should trust her expertise. He did not care to remember the nitty-gritties—what drugs were used and for what purpose, what my estradiol levels were, what my FSH level was, what his own sperm count was, what the cost of the treatment was. He had no clue.

~

It was day seven of the first IVF cycle. I went to the fertility clinic in the morning for my shots and blood tests and reached office at eleven, an embarrassing two hours late. A couple of stares and raised eyebrows followed me to my workstation. Just as I was settling down to edit a presentation, my phone rang. Sini was calling to say that the results of the blood tests had come in; I had to go back to the hospital for another round of supplementary injections. It was only noon. I walked with trepidation to my manager's cabin, explained the situation and asked if I could leave at one. She said 'yes' unhesitatingly, but I nearly bit my tongue making a request that sounded so outlandish and unreasonable even to my own ears. My manager was in the know about my IVF cycle and had agreed to the leeway I needed. But there was no explanation to offer my peers, who must have wondered what was going on. An hour later I slung my laptop bag and handbag on my shoulders and walked out; the same stares and raised eyebrows followed me to the parking lot. I had spent barely two hours at my desk, the rest of my working day vanished in running between office and hospital.

In the evening, when Ranjith sauntered in, his time and body untouched by IVF, I was seething from the frustration of being the sole bearer of the IVF cross. He dropped his backpack on the sofa, went to the bedroom, changed and then came into the kitchen. He picked up a plate from the rack and helped himself to dinner.

'How was your day?' he asked casually.

I said nothing.

'*Enthu petti*? Something's wrong?' He tried again.

He put the plate down and came close to me.

'What's wrong? Tell me. I am no mind reader.'

I sighed.

'I can't do this any more. I drove four hours and sixty kilometres today between the hospital and office to have six needles inserted inside and three vials of blood drawn. I couldn't get one thing done at work. And all you have to do is come home in the evening, throw your bag on the sofa and ask, "How was your day?" That's how easy this is for you.'

'Why? What happened?'

'You knew I was going to the clinic in the morning. You could have called me to find out how it went. Better still, you could have come with me. How come this thought never crosses your mind?'

'OK, OK. I am sorry. I didn't know you had a rough day. What do you want me to do?'

'Ranjith, I am sick of telling you what to do. You are not a child and I am not your mother to give you instructions. I expect you to act of your own volition and bring some involvement into this process. You can't just stand in a corner and watch from a distance all the time.'

'Do you have any idea how helpless I feel watching you go through this? But there is nothing I can do to contribute. That's the way biology is. If I could take a pill or an injection on your behalf, I would have done it in a split second. But unfortunately there is nothing for me to do. Is it my fault?'

'No, it's not your fault. But you have made peace with it so quickly and closed that chapter. I don't see you do anything to make up for it in any other way. You are not even there for me emotionally.'

'That's not fair. I trust you. You are an independent, capable woman and I know you are doing the best you can. If there is anything you want me to do specifically, just tell me.'

'You can't say "I trust you" and wash your hands of this. That's very convenient. I am doing everything alone. I take responsibility for the clinic, the doctor, the procedure, the treatment protocol; I go through the ultrasounds, injections, blood test, pills, while you can barely tell the difference between sperm and egg. If at all I need anything from you, it has to be spelled out. Do you have any idea how alone I feel?'

'See. I am a guy who looks at the big picture. As far as I am concerned there is no need to take all this "responsibility", fill yourself with knowledge from the Internet and obsess over every data point. Our goal is to have a baby and we have appointed a specialist doctor for this. Just let medicine do its job and let's hope that everything turns out well. It's as simple as that.'

'As usual, you oversimplify everything.'

'And you overcomplicate everything.'

'So it's *my* fault now? I am the one going through this shit and you have the gall to tell me that I am overreacting.'

'No, I didn't say that . . .'

The argument stretched until it reached stalemate and fizzled out. I went to sleep, wiped out from the emotional battles. Ranjith stationed himself in front of the TV to watch football being played in some corner of the world where it was still day.

There was some merit in what he said but there was no way I could adopt a dispassionate and stoic stance, as he had. This was all happening inside my body and I did not have the luxury of forgetting even for a single waking hour that I was going through fertility treatment. Besides, I was someone who did endless research on Google about every subatomic particle in my life. I hated going into any situation without prior information. This is how I planned a holiday: bookmarking and memorizing blogs on the destination, shortlisting tourist guides, surveying friends, neighbours and colleagues who had already been to the same place; studying images, watching YouTube videos, poring through answers on Quora . . . to craft a carefully curated itinerary. I would also research the geopolitical situation, weather pattern and cultural ethos of the region. If it was a foreign country I would query the time taken to clear immigration, customs, and look up airline and airport rankings. By the time I was ready to board the aircraft I'd have gathered enough material for an MPhil dissertation. I couldn't just get up one day, decide to go someplace, take my bags and leave, acting on a moment of impulse and spontaneity. That would be a nightmare, not a holiday. And my obsessive, compulsive, controlling nature collided with Ranjith's calm, easy-going, take-it-in-your-stride approach nowhere more violently than during this infertility treatment—my overwhelming craziness set off against his underwhelming coolness.

Ranjith was absent for three out of the four IUIs. On a couple of occasions he came in and gave his semen sample on the previous day of the IUIs when it was convenient for him. We thawed the frozen sample on the day of the procedure. For IVF, I told him over the course of many arguments that his fence-sitting approach wouldn't do. He had to make himself available for as many hospital visits as he could. He agreed and made efforts to give more time. During the first IVF cycle his involvement exceeded that at all the previous IUIs. Yet his enthusiasm never matched mine; he was always slightly detached. We had our fair share of fights on this topic. He never understood my anxiety and I never understood his lack of it. After a point, I realized that I was just alienating him further by constantly accusing him of being disinterested.

But it continued to be a sore wound that would flare up every now and then.

~

On our first holiday after marriage, we had booked into a homestay in a coffee plantation in Coorg. There were a couple of other families staying in the same plantation. One night we sat around a bonfire enjoying the impromptu performances put up by the children from the other cottages. After the children finished, someone decided adults too must pitch in. Each of us had to take turns to sing, dance or display some other non-talent. I sank in my chair, wishing I had a cloak of invisibility to put on. I insisted that Ranjith would sing on my behalf. The others did not relent. One of the guests, a soft-spoken man in his early forties, set out to correct my notions of marriage.

'I am going to tell you something that is true for all marriages. Each partner has to pull his or her own weight in the relationship. You must hold your own. One person cannot be the substitute for the other.'

That night I still managed to dodge the bullet by asking Ranjith to stand in for me at the campfire. But this nugget of wisdom stayed with me, and all through my marriage I tried to enforce it. I understood the man's words to mean that everything in marriage is a 50:50 partnership. I would put in my share and expect an equal share in return. When I didn't get my 50 per cent back it was frustrating; I would launch into offence mode, activating a cycle of arguments, accusations and silences. I felt perpetually victimized and Ranjith felt like a perpetual target of blame.

When I look back now, it feels immature and shortsighted. No marriage, or for that matter no relationship, is always an equally divided proposition. Sometimes I had to give 80 per cent and could expect only 20 per cent from the other. And sometimes it was the opposite. Fertility treatment would always be an unbalanced, lopsided equation, and biology was the culprit in some ways. But I had to remind myself that Ranjith made up for his absences here in other ways, and for the sake of our marriage and happiness I had to divert my attention to what he did rather than what he did not. He was my biggest cheerleader, egging me on to dream bigger and higher at work, a solver of all the daily riddles and puzzles I brought back home from office. He was needlessly generous, pampering me with lavish gifts on birthdays, anniversaries and Valentine's. He ceded control regarding most practicalities, letting me rejoice in deciding which gadgets to buy, how to decorate our home, whom to invite for dinner and where to holiday. He stayed in the background most of the time, stepping in only when invited. He was in many ways my safety net and my springboard.

Ranjith was a classic Piscean, shifty and slippery like a fish. It was impossible to pin him down to any one pursuit. He did not want to get subsumed by the infertility issue, and he glided in and out of that universe. Sometimes there. Sometimes not. That was *his* survival instinct. In an ideal world we would have waded through this shoulder to shoulder, hand in hand. But instead, we travelled through the darkness in our own two different and separate ways.

~

The results of the AMH test came after fifteen days. It took longer than other blood tests because it required specialized equipment and was outsourced to a speciality lab.

Sini called to inform me that the report had arrived at the IVF clinic. At my next visit I picked it up from the reception area and ran through the pages. My heart sank several hundred feet. The AMH level was 2.35; it had fallen a whole point from 3.4. I was standing on the threshold of acceptability, one foot dangling outside. At this rate, we didn't have much time left before the door closed on me.

Dr Leela, however, seemed unperturbed. 'It is still within the range. We can start the second IVF cycle next month.'

8

Leaving Home

Ranjith likes to call Trivandrum 'capital city'. When I tease him about his choice of clothes or taste in cinema, he responds with, 'You are from the capital city. I am from the countryside. What do I know?' We both laugh because he knows too well that the Trivandrum in which I grew up hardly fits the bill of 'capital city'. It had none of the glamour, expanse or pull of capital cities. Peopled mostly by government employees, bank officers, teachers and the odd artist or writer, Trivandrum was actually more of a small town, offering a modest middle-class life—safe, neat, green, with reasonably good schools, colleges and hospitals. Most youngsters of my generation dreamt of moving to Bangalore, Chennai, or at the very least Kochi, once they were old enough. By the time I was in my teens I was acutely aware of the 'smallness' of where I came from. I resented its lack of cosmopolitanism, the absence of the big-city vibe and opportunities.

It was the late 1990s when cable TV had just penetrated the so-called tier-two and tier-three cities in India and channels like MTV and Channel V were beaming images of young, modern, westernized Indian youth into our homes. My friends and I gaped at the students who poured out of colleges in Bombay and Delhi. We noted that the young girls wore jeans as an everyday unthinking choice, while Trivandrum had only one shop that even *sold* jeans for women. And the meagre pairs of jeans we owned were only worn in solidarity with other girlfriends to avoid standing out too much. In the metros, boys and girls interacted freely, shaking hands, backslapping and hugging each other, blurring what we saw as lines of propriety. Where we grew up, only brothers and sisters could be so publicly demonstrative without attracting disapproval. In the cities, weekend entertainment reeled around parties, discotheques and pub crawls, while in our town hardly anyone stepped out after dusk, weekend or weekday. Television was a window to a world that was so alien, yet so desirable. I, certainly, felt I wanted a part of that world. That's when I began dreaming of moving to one of the large, busy, crowded, constantly-moving, never-sleeping cities. I longed to be lost in one of them. As a young girl growing up in the 'capital city', I couldn't wait to leave.

~

The class ten boards fiasco proved to be precisely the psychotherapy I needed. It was the hare-and-tortoise lesson of my life. I exorcised the sloth and overconfidence of the hare and imbibed the focus, stamina and steady pace of the tortoise. I drew up elaborate timetables, put up inspirational quotes in front of my desk and gulped down endless caffeine to pull all-nighters. From one end of the spectrum I swung to the other, now too scared to let up lest I should fall behind again. At the end of the pre-degree programme, I found a place among the university toppers. The ignominy of my class ten results was erased and replaced with instant celebrity.

A close-up photo of my face appeared on the front page of the city newspapers the next day along those of other subject toppers. TV channels carried my byte during the evening news bulletin. Amma went delirious attending to the continuous stream of visitors dropping in or calling to congratulate me. Achan bragged to all and sundry about how he had supported my decision to pursue the arts and thereby propelled this success. My fifteen-year-old brother's only occupation that day was with the one hundred laddoos my mother bought from G.G. Bakery for distribution. Neither envious nor overawed by the attention his sibling was getting, he trained his focus on the laddoos.

The success was a reinforcement of the lessons extrapolated from failure. The fanfare, attention and rewards made me conclude that this was going to be my approach to life. Set a goal. Achieve the goal. Move on to the next goal. Determination, discipline and hard work would see me through life's obstacles. There was nothing wrong with the formula; it was largely helpful in navigating educational and professional aims. It worked beautifully, until I brought my goal-oriented, process-driven, bulleted and numbered template to something as frustratingly complex and enigmatic as human biology. Biology laughed out loud at the rules I had set for life.

~

Having secured top marks, the thought crossed my mind that I could apply to a leading college in Chennai or Bangalore for an undergraduate degree in English literature. Amma's cousin who lived in Chennai even mailed me application forms from the prominent colleges in the city. But my parents wanted me to wait until postgraduation to move out; this they deemed was the appropriate life-stage at which to send a young woman out into the world on her own. A male cousin, about the same age as I was and nurturing the same dreams, left Trivandrum soon after class twelve to pursue a degree in hotel management in Chennai. No one wondered if it was the right age for him.

I made some simpering protests and brought up my cousin's example a couple of times, but mostly let go without a fight. I was at a delicate, unsure age myself, not confident enough to challenge my parent's worldly wisdom. Besides, leaving home was a frightening prospect and I lapped up an excuse to defer it. So I stayed on in Trivandrum and rejoined the same girls-only college for their undergraduate programme.

It was one of the best colleges in town but the university syllabus was woefully out of date. When I joined a national-level institution for a postgraduate programme later, I passed out on discovering terms like 'postcolonialism', 'gender studies' or 'Dalit writing', because in our curriculum we stayed loyal to the Victorian age, making allowance only for the odd Indian writer in English. The course did not demand critical analysis, additional readings or any kind of serious student input. You could whizz through three years of the undergraduate programme without framing an original sentence. Quite a few of us didn't even bother reading the actual textbooks. There were companion guides available to every text. You could just memorize the sample questions and answers and coolly ace the exams. Only later did I realize how much I had been shortchanged by my education. It took two full semesters of the master's course for me to even follow the discussion in class and produce a worthy assignment, to understand what it means to 'problematize a text', 'to turn an argument on its head'. Hell! To even make an argument. For the first time in my life, after almost fifteen years of schooling and college, I was required to think and write independently. *Where are the guides when you really need them?*

But the college itself was close to the heart and the setting for many fond memories. The campus was located on the outskirts of the city. There was nothing architecturally unique or historically relevant about it—a series of rectangular buildings assigned to different subject groups. But the location was born out of an urban artist's imagination. It stood at the confluence of a railway line, an airfield and a beach. A railway track curved around the perimeter of the campus and our entry and exit from college was constantly punctuated by the schedule of passing trains. Every day in the afternoon, we waited for the Kanyakumari-bound Island Express to thunder past the crossing before the college gates were opened. If the train was delayed, so were we.

On the other side of the road was the tail end of the airport runway. From the bus stop our eyes often followed the trajectory of aircraft touching down and taking off, bringing the aura of faraway places to the placidity of the quiet town. In class, we waited for these sounds—the chug of a train or the roar of an aircraft—to drown out a professor and provide a few seconds of relief in a seemingly interminable lecture.

The college was an extension of the convent schools that many of us came from. Ornate wrought iron gates guarded us from the outside world. It was an Abhimanyu-and-Chakravyuh scenario. You could walk into the college at any time, but you could walk out only at the end of the day when classes were over. By three in the afternoon girls would begin to hustle near the gate to board one of the KSRTC (government service) buses parked outside. The security guard brandished a long stick to keep the girls in line and to make sure that no one bolted before he decided it was time. Some spirited girls of course smoothly subverted the tall towers and armed guard by not entering the campus at all. They got off the buses that brought them to college in the morning and hopped onto the steeds parked outside for a day out in town with their suitors.

Political parties were not allowed to operate inside the college. This was an anomaly in Kerala, where colleges are known for the polarizing and strident politics of student unions. But we were sheltered from these rivalries in the breezy, apolitical climate of the campus. There was a college students' union, whose primary mandate was to conduct annual day events and other cultural programmes. The most critical responsibility of the arts club secretary was to invite a celebrity—preferably a young heartthrob movie actor—for the inauguration of the club. It was a cloistered environment and had its drawbacks, but it was also liberating to inhabit a girls-only universe. It was safe, protected and fun. We could drop the extra armour required in the buses and streets on our way back home which were happy hunting grounds for sexual predators.

I have lost count of the number of times and the number of ways in which I have been molested. Flashing penises, fumbling hands that poked me from the seat behind, deliberate brushes against my chest in an overflowing bus, unsolicited opinion on the size of my breasts or the shape of my buttocks . . . As a child who started commuting alone by public transport at the age of thirteen, I have seen and endured more than I should have. And every time I heeded my mother's advice and stayed quiet, notwithstanding the burning in my face and the hammering in my chest. 'Ignore it.' 'Don't make a scene.' 'Talking back makes it worse,' she had told me. No, it doesn't. But it was very late before I saw the harm in that counsel.

~

College gave me my best friend. At the end of the first day of classes I came home and wept. I told Amma despondently, 'I don't like college. I don't think I will ever make any friends.' Sara told me later that she too went home and cried on the shoulders of her elder sister. Her sister rolled her eyes and said, 'It's only been a day. Give it some time.' The next day we caught each other's attention, and our college lives went from tragic black-and-white to a joyous explosion of technicolour. Meeting her was like finding my 'cool' twin. She was tall and lean, just like me, but she was also warm, friendly and vivacious. I was quiet, reserved and nerdy. She was Miss Congeniality, and I was the wallflower. But we fell in love with each other. She introduced me to boy bands and Hollywood films. I created my first-ever email account on her computer, sitting in her room, seeing it as an amusement, never imagining it would be of any use. I had my first-ever facial in the same room, spending three hours on a Saturday afternoon having my face rubbed, massaged and steamed to her lively commentary. We spent many sleepless nights within the same walls, weaving dreams and schemes for the future. We asked again and again the same questions—When will I fall in love? Whom will I fall in love with? Will anything come of our dreams? What will change? What will remain the same?

The coolest hangout on our teen landscape was a bakery called Ambrosia. Ambrosia differentiated itself from its counterparts by offering pizzas, burgers and sandwiches, apart from the standard fare of puffs, cutlets and Indian sweets. Their fresh cream cakes were the fanciest in town. With high kitchen stools, bar-like counter tops and hanging lights, it almost pulled off a hip vibe. It was *the* place in Trivandrum for the with-it crowd. Being there was the high point of our social life and reserved for special occasions. After one such lavish celebration, Sara and I made a pact that we would meet in Ambrosia on our birthdays every year. Well, like most college pacts, that didn't even last till the next birthday!

Last year, after twenty years, I caught up with Sara in Ambrosia. We had succeeded in sustaining our relationship, despite the four cities, two countries, jobs, husbands and children that came between us. Now we could indulge ourselves without worrying about measly allowances, but we ordered only lemon tea and garlic bread (and that too, a single portion). At thirty-seven, you know way too much about snacking, empty calories and nutritional value to fall for the pastries.

We vented on a range of topics—our non-existent careers, messy marriages, disapproving in-laws and wayward children. It was the kind of animated and heartfelt conversation that you can only have with a girlfriend from the same college and the same city in which you grew up. Our voices clashed and collided, unable to contain the excitement of being seventeen again. Twenty years melted away in a matter of ninety minutes. Everything changes. Everything remains the same. If only I had known this when I was so desperate to snap my ties with Trivandrum.

~

In the final year of the undergraduate programme, I started plotting my escape from the small pond. My parents made peace with the fact that I was determined to fly out of their nest. I sat for entrance exams to institutions across the country for a master's in English literature and made it through most of them. I chose an institute in Hyderabad from the ones that chose me. The institute offered an interdisciplinary format and the freedom to build depth in a sub-discipline vis-a-vis a broad degree in literature. I thought it would give me the right inputs for a strong CV and a better take-off in the job market. I didn't have the faintest intention of coming back to Trivandrum; this was my exit once and for all from the small town. Hyderabad was also geographically and culturally ideal. Not too far, not too near. Not too hip like Bangalore or too old-school like Chennai. It had art, culture, history and biriyani. The decision was made.

After a month of shopping, exchanging farewell gifts and letters and attending farewell parties, I was ready to leave. To embrace a life of freedom, choice and achievement. I was all of twenty. The night before I boarded the train that would take me to Secunderabad, I sat in my room and surveyed my two suitcases filled with salwar kameez, a pair of jeans and three newly bought tops, some books, a kettle, a portable table lamp, a photo frame, a Walkman and a few cassettes. A wave of sadness washed over me, and I cried copiously into my pillow. I didn't sleep that night. The next morning, as I bid goodbye to Achan through the window of the sleeper-class compartment, the tightness and firmness of his handshake left me crushed. The train reached Ernakulam, five and a half hours away, before I could swallow the lump in my throat and summon the composure to speak. As the train drew further and further away from Trivandrum and then Kerala itself, life as I knew it until then started to fade. It was the first unravelling of my life. The wound caused by that severing never quite healed.

In Hyderabad I dreamt of my city every night for months. I walked through the streets, negotiating the familiar winds and turns, enjoying the sudden bursts of green, sliding in and out of familiar spaces—our house, my college, my room. I bottled the city up like a fragrance, uncorking and relishing the smell every night. The sum total of everything I knew and held dear in this world resided in that city. I missed its innocence, its warmth, its languor. It took years before I could call another place home. Even though I moved out of Trivandrum, Trivandrum never left me.

9

Grades Don't Matter

I always thought the worst thing that can happen in an IVF cycle is failing to get pregnant. That is, until I signed up for one. With the first cycle, I realized that an IVF cycle is not a litmus test, a single-step, red-or-blue kind of process that determines if you have made it or not. It's a multi-part, sequential obstacle race. There are warped walls to climb over, muddy waters to wade through, and barbed wire to crawl under. The pregnancy test is the very last and relatively minor hurdle in this. Before that I must clear the laborious stages of ovarian stimulation, egg retrieval and embryo transfer. The uterus must produce enough follicles to warrant an egg pick-up and the resultant embryos must qualify for embryo transfer. And finally, the endometrial lining should be thick enough to receive the waiting embryos. If I didn't make the grade at any one of these intervening steps, I would be out of the chase. In fact, if there was a thing even worse than failing the pregnancy test, that was not being able to get to it. I concluded that to complete a full-length IVF cycle—

with all its mud pits, rocky trails and slippery slides—was an achievement in itself.

~

We began the second IVF cycle in December 2012 by throwing down the gauntlet to my ovaries. Dr Leela cranked up the dose of ovarian stimulating medicines hoping to wrest a higher number of eggs from my body's reserve. I stopped by at the clinic on my way to work and took three shots daily. A few days in, we also began blood tests to monitor the rising levels of various hormones, and transvaginal ultrasounds to gauge the development of follicles.

IVF involves goading your ovaries into delivering an extreme level of performance by pumping in a copious volume of hormones. The goal is to trigger the release of maybe five, ten or twenty eggs from one cycle instead of the usual one or two. One of the fallouts of this 'shock and awe' treatment is that it puts you at risk of ovarian hyperstimulation syndrome; your ovaries overreact to the medication, causing them to become swollen and painful, inducing other symptoms such as bloating, abdominal pain, nausea and weight gain. My reproductive system, however, had had the opposite problem so far; it reacted too leisurely to the drugs. The estradiol levels climbed slowly, and my ovaries were tight-fisted about releasing eggs from their home.

This time, however, my uterus hit the right notes from the word go. Follicles grew in number and size as the cycle progressed, and by day twelve I had thirteen fully grown follicles, one of which I believed carried the germ of my yet-to-be-born child. This was more than double the number I had in the first IVF cycle. There was another patient going through stimulation at the same time in the clinic. I heard from Sini that she had twenty-three follicles!

I never really made any friends in the clinic. Everyone is on a different schedule so you don't meet the same people each time. And while my pregnancy was taking longer to happen, a lot of others who started out with me got pregnant faster or moved to another clinic or stopped treatment altogether. Only one time I ran into someone I knew from my office. We acknowledged each other's presence and shared a few stale pleasantries, but it was very clear that there was no scope to go beyond that. There is a very thick veil of shame that hangs above most who enter the IVF clinic.

On the follicles front, I did not top the IVF class, but I did not fare too badly either. Thirteen was a respectable number. The thickness of my endometrial lining was an optimal 10 mm. The day of the trigger shot, I felt quietly secure and confident going into egg retrieval.

Egg retrieval was my favourite day of IVF. It was done in the operating theatre under anaesthesia. A needle was inserted through the vagina to drain out the fluid from the follicles (the eggs are found floating in the fluid), which was then collected in test tubes and transferred to a laboratory. I looked forward to sedation; in the middle of the cycle, it offered an escape from the constant worrying about the achievements of my reproductive system. I even enjoyed the drowsy half a day or so that followed general anaesthesia when I drifted in a daze in the obscure regions between reality and dream.

That day when my eyes opened, I had been shifted out of the operating theatre into the recovery room. I lay on a bed against a wall, partitioned by white polyester curtains on three sides. Sini, my friend-cum-nurse, was hovering about in the clinic. I asked her about the number of eggs retrieved.

She said, 'Eight.'

'*Eight?*' I thought I hadn't heard her correctly.

'Yes, eight.'

'Just *eight?*'

Just eight eggs from thirteen follicles? What happened to the others? Even in my semi-conscious state I had enough clarity to know that eight was not a good number. In the last ultrasound before the trigger shot, I had thirteen handsome follicles, which should have released at least ten to twelve eggs. But we had only *eight* now. What had gone wrong?

In the first IVF cycle I had six eggs which led to *one* grade-A embryo. With eight eggs this time, I could expect to have maybe *two or three* high-quality embryos. The second cycle was only marginally better than the first, despite the higher dose of drugs. This also meant that if this cycle did not result in a pregnancy, I would have to stomach another round of ovarian stimulation. I was counting on having half a dozen embryos so that we could freeze the surplus ones for future use, maybe even to have a second child. This would spare me the woes of stimulation with the fifty thousand injections, ultrasounds and blood tests, not to mention the added costs. But my uterus was not in the mood to cut me any slack.

This cycle had been coming together quite well until now and seemed poised to result in a positive pregnancy test. But when I heard that number my hopes crashed. Another patient might have been happy to have eight eggs or might not even have appreciated the difference between producing eight eggs and twelve eggs, but for someone like me who was so focused on the fine print, it registered as yet another middling performance and yet another mishap in the making.

My mind was still foggy from anaesthesia. Unsure if I was awake or dreaming, I concluded that I must be asleep and, in the safety of my sleep, I thought it was okay to let go as no one was watching. All the heartache accrued over the years tumbled out and I cried a helpless cry. Not just for the eight eggs, but for all the things that had gone right and wrong in treatment, for the months and years of seesawing hope and loss of hope, for my husband waiting outside oblivious to my cries, for being denied even a tiny scrap of good fortune.

'What's wrong? Is something hurting?' Sini was at my bed, confused and concerned.

I realized I was shedding actual tears; I was not crying in a dream. This was real and visible to others. I felt embarrassed.

'Only eight, just eight,' I mumbled through the sobs in explanation.

'Don't worry, you only need one. That is seven too many,' she replied dismissively.

I had heard this line too many times for it to leave an impression.

Sini said a few more things to pacify me, then seeing it made no difference gave up and went back to her chores.

I turned to the side facing the wall and spent the next three hours crying. I mourned the too-few eggs, the too-many cycles, and the too-little payoff. In the flimsy solitude of that hospital bed screened by white curtains, I mourned all the injustices in my life that caused varying degrees of hurt. Two extra eggs would have made all the difference.

~

It was a Wednesday. I was back at my desk after the day off for egg retrieval. I brought a cup of tea from the pantry one floor below and sat down to organize my inbox. In twenty minutes I had brought the count of unread emails down from thirty-four to four. Few things are as gratifying as archiving emails. Around noon, I got a call on my mobile phone from the IVF clinic. It was Praveen Kumar, the embryologist. Praveen was reserved and serious, giving the impression of someone who had no interest in anything outside his laboratory. He was content to deal only with pipettes, petri dishes and incubators. Even though we had seen each other many times in the clinic we had never exchanged greetings.

Praveen was calling to share my report card: How many eggs had fertilized? What was their grade? Once the eggs are extricated from the woman's body, an intra-cytoplasmic sperm injection or ICSI is performed. Each egg is individually combined with the sperm to achieve fertilization. Dr Leela chose ICSI over letting the egg and sperm meet naturally in a petri dish because she felt it was more efficient and had a greater success rate of fertilization.

My mind was calm and lucid by now, and I awaited the information with studied indifference. The previous day's tears had untangled my coiled-up heart and reset my expectations from the cycle back to zero. Another crash and burn, I thought.

Praveen introduced himself and spoke in a soft, neutral tone without giving any hint of whether the news was good or bad. As if he had no insight into what was at stake for the person at the other end of the line.

He said, 'Seven out of the eight eggs have fertilized.'

'Okay.' *Seven?*

'They are all of excellent quality.'

'Okay.' *What?*

'We can plan to do a day-five transfer with two of the best-looking ones!'

I nearly jumped out of my seat in disbelief. *What? Seven good embryos? And a day-five transfer?* So what if I had only eight eggs? All but one had fertilized and that was an excellent ratio of conversion from egg to embryo. I had passed with flying colours. I did the mental equivalent of several pole vaults before landing on my feet.

I thanked Praveen profusely and quickly rang Ranjith to give him the news. I stood at my desk repeating the things Praveen had just finished telling me. *Who knew eggs could make me so deliriously happy?*

We turned up five days after the egg retrieval for the embryo transfer. The mood at the clinic was relaxed and upbeat. One of the nurses had just returned from a trip home to Kerala and had brought several home-made delicacies. Sini invited me into the consultation room where everyone had gathered for tea and snacks. My extended bawling of the other day had moved everyone at the clinic. They were as overjoyed as I was to learn that I had seven healthy embryos this time. The DHEA tablets had done some magic after all.

The embryo transfer took place in the same operating theatre as the egg retrieval, but this time without anaesthesia. Two grade-A blastocysts were placed inside my uterus in a procedure mimicking IUI, and the remaining five embryos were stored in the freezer, to be used for ensuing cycles, *if it came to that.*

Blastocyst is a stage in embryo development which is reached typically after five or six days of fertilization. At this stage, the embryo is a spherical cluster of two hundred cells and looks like the microscopic version of a crater-ridden lunar object. A blastocyst is pegged with higher chances of implantation because it is at a more advanced embryonic stage. The grades indicate their quality, with 'A' being excellent quality and 'C' being very poor quality. Grades are assigned to embryos in an IVF cycle to aid decision-making. It helps the doctor assess the viability of the embryo and the potential for success. By looking at the number, form, texture and appearance of the cells, the doctor arrives at embryo maturity and quality. The better the quality of the embryo, the more it is likely to result in a live-term birth.

In the first IVF cycle I had only three embryos. One was grade-A, another grade-B and the third grade-C. Dr Leela dropped all three inside me in the wild hope that one of them would sprout. The grade-B and C embryos had a grim forecast, but they were just bundled along with the premium embryo. But this time I had two grade-A embryos and one was a hatching blastocyst[1]—meaning, they were quite close to flawless. There was an unspoken sense among everyone in the clinic that this cycle was going to be the clincher.

The transfer took only ten minutes, but I had to rest in the clinic for three to four hours after that. By two in the afternoon I was ready to be discharged. I went home with the hospital dossier, which contained the discharge summary, prescription and, most precious of all, photos of the embryos.

---

[1] 'A hatching blastocyst is a developing embryo (at around five days after fertilization) that is hatching out of its protective coating, known as the zona pellucida.' (Source: https://www.fertilitysmarts.com/definition/1215/hatching-blastocyst, accessed in August 2020.)

They were greyish-bluish grainy images of orb-like structures. I gloated over them for a long time, comparing them with samples from the Internet. I was already calculating the pros and cons of a life with twins.

The beta hCG test was scheduled two weeks from the embryo transfer. There were various medicines and injections to support the upcoming pregnancy. Besides that, there were three directives: No travelling long distance. Normal food. Intake of plenty of fluids. I stayed true to these, but did not observe any further precautions, except in the matter of driving.

On the cut-throat streets of Bangalore with bumper-to-bumper traffic, the unspoken credo is, don't give an inch. If you give an inch you will be behind by a mile. Since I had learnt to drive here I swore by this, daily exhorting my 2006 black Wagon-R to go beyond the limits set by its maker. I did not slow down at any orange light; it was a sign to cross the intersection before the light turned red. I didn't see the difference between overtaking from the right or the left of the car in front. I honked mercilessly and raised my eyebrows and hands at drivers whom I felt were stalling my progress. But now, given my quasi-pregnant status (two embryos had been planted inside my body), I decided to adopt a more mellow approach. Perhaps an inch here, an inch there wouldn't do any harm.

~

A week after the embryo transfer, I felt mild cramping in my abdomen, as if a tiny creature was burrowing a hole inside my womb. I could distinctly feel the scratching. Then I had a vivid early morning dream in which I was giving birth to twins. By now I was certain that *this time* I was pregnant. I couldn't wait to take a home pregnancy test (HPT) and confirm my hunch.

Doctors warn against taking HPTs during an IVF cycle as you are on supplementary hCG injections which can skew the results, leading to false positives.

The hCG hormone can be detected in an HPT only twelve to fourteen days after fertilization. The levels have to be high and concentrated enough to show up in urine droplets. So if you take an HPT too soon you could get a false negative. The safest thing to do is to wait for a beta hCG test, in which a blood sample is used to measure the exact level of the hormone in the body. Any value above 25 mIU/mL is generally considered a sign of pregnancy. But I was disinclined towards anything sensible.

I waited for ten days after the embryo transfer (which meant about fifteen days after fertilization) and took my first HPT. It was negative. It was disheartening, but maybe it was too early, I told myself. The Indian brands don't reveal the sensitivity of the test (the lowest level of hCG that the test can measure) and just ask you to wait at least a week after a missed period to be absolutely sure, though it is quite common to get a positive result one or two days after a missed period. I was only fifteen days past fertilization and it was a grey zone.

But in the corners of my heart I didn't entirely buy the 'it's-too-early' hypothesis because these testing guidelines made sense in the case of natural conception where the woman isn't sure when fertilization has taken place, if at all it has. In my case I knew exactly when fertilization had taken place and how many embryos were inside the womb. The only question left to answer was if they had implanted. Implantation typically occurs within six to ten days of egg retrieval or fertilization and the foetus starts producing the hCG hormone soon after that. So if the embryos had embedded themselves in my uterus I should have got a positive HPT by now, as it was almost a week past the implantation window. Maybe they implanted late, I told myself. But even that wasn't convincing because one of the embryos was already hatching out of its outer shell when the transfer took place.

I waited three more days and took another HPT. It was negative again. This time I couldn't believe my eyes. I held the test under sunlight, shook it down like a mercury thermometer, left it alone for some time and then checked again. The test did not yield; the second line was stubbornly absent. My understanding of pregnancy testing told me that if this cycle had worked, by now the HPT would have been positive. It was now eighteen days past fertilization and there was still no sign of the hCG hormone in my body. The writing on the wall was in all caps and bold. The embryos had failed to implant.

I went into shock. How could this have failed? I had two *grade-A blastocysts* transferred on day five. It was a textbook case, a classic example of embryo perfection, a reproductive specialist's dream come true. But the star embryos, backed by science and research to grow into chubby-cheeked gurgling babies, had failed at the very first step. They had turned back, unwilling to travel any further.

Dr Preetha's words echoed in my ears. Dr Preetha was the fifty-something second-in-charge doctor in the IVF clinic. She doubled up as the unofficial agony aunt and therapist, taking the time to listen to patients, often sharing her own experiences from a long career in medicine, pointing out examples from other patient histories or even breaking down some of the scientific details which Dr Leela left unexplained.

She always told me, 'Biology is not a precise science like maths. In maths two plus two is always equal to four. In biology, a grade-A embryo may fail to implant inside the uterine lining. At the same time, a grade-C embryo might lead to a healthy baby. So, you never know.' It was an incredibly inspiring comment to hear when you had a grade-C embryo, but a terribly depressing one when you had the grade-A one.

That morning, with the second negative HPT lying in the dustbin, I buried my faith in medical science. What was the purpose of these grades and decorations? What good had come of them? Medicine was no better than a capricious, irrational despot doling out rewards or denying them. In the end, nothing mattered—not the embryos, not their grades, not the signs and symptoms. It was all down to the lines on my forehead.

What I didn't know then is that embryo grading is assessment of quality at face value. It doesn't tell you anything about the internal make-up of the embryo, if there are any genetic defects or chromosomal abnormalities. It was an imperfect and indeterminate system, but that's all we had. And besides, I knew, conditioned by my education, that the next time and every time, given a choice, I would put my money and faith on a grade-A embryo over a grade-C one.

I realized that the worst kind of IVF cycle is the one where you sail through all the preliminary tasks, scoring perfect tens and yet fall short at the grand finale. Yes, completing something as taxing and draining as an IVF cycle *is* an achievement. At the end of the IVF month, I had logged fifty injections, four ultrasounds, four rounds of blood tests, general anaesthesia and up to twenty-five pills *daily* during the two-week wait. But you can't draw much comfort from that kind of achievement. In IVF, there are no consolation prizes.

I drove to office that Friday and acted out the part of a fully functional human being capable of coherent speech and productive work. But my mind was engulfed in an opaque haze; it was trapped in a senseless blur. The signs had been so strong this time and yet I was once again deceived by my body. How could I trust such a treacherous instrument again? Would I ever see a positive pregnancy test in my life?

'Let's go out of town for the weekend. A change of scene is needed,' said Ranjith over the phone.

He had called at noon to check on me. When I informed him in the morning that another IVF boat had sunk without a trace, he didn't react. He was his usual stoic self, only offering his ear to soak up my despondency.

'Yes. You find the place and do the booking. I don't care where we go.'

He picked me up after work and we drove to a rustic village-style resort on the outskirts of Bangalore. There was no TV or AC. Only sattvic food and very few guests. When we walked in late Friday evening, our room was filled with the smoke and smell of incense. It was precisely the salve that our wounded selves needed. Over the next two days I took long baths, read a book, watched a Malayalam movie on our laptop and slowly found my way back to wholeness.

By Monday, all the blurring, melting parts had solidified, and cohesion restored. I still had to take the beta hCG test for official confirmation, but since the result was known I was unconcerned. This cycle was a closed chapter. The only saving grace was that we still had five frozen embryos and could make at least two more attempts.

As I drove back home during rush hour on Monday evening I channelled all my pent-up roadside aggression. I raced over potholes, changed lanes abruptly and jammed the accelerator and brake pedals in careless succession to get past all things human and man-made that stood between me and my apartment. It didn't matter. I was not pregnant. I might as well reach home fast.

10

The Keeper of Secrets

On Tuesday morning I went to the IVF clinic to give a blood sample for the beta hCG test.

While leaving home earlier that day, Ranjith had asked me wistfully one final time, 'Do we have *any* reason for hope?'

'No,' I said, firmly.

'Should I come with you to the clinic for the test?'

'No. You carry on. We already know the result. This is just a formality.'

I killed all remnants of hope floating in the atmosphere, flattening the graph before setting out for the hospital.

At the clinic, I sat on the chair arranged perpendicular to a table in the nurse's station and stretched my arm out. Sini was her usual jovial self. When the needle went under my skin, she said teasingly, 'We have marked you at 99.5 per cent.' I did not have the heart to tell her that I had already taken an HPT and it was negative. I smiled and laughed, careful not to let my anguish rise to the surface. She would find out soon enough, I thought, as I walked to my car in the parking to drive to office.

The clinic was expected to share the result by noon. My colleague Arun and I had lunch at the neighbouring campus of an IT company. They had a large, sprawling cafeteria with plenty of counters and cuisines. The din of the space allowed us to share office gossip, complain about our colleagues, and vent, fearless of being overheard. Lunch in the cafeteria provided the much-needed mid-day release of pressure. Around one, just as we were walking back to our own building, my phone rang. I signalled to Arun to carry on and moved aside to take the call.

I heard Dr Preetha's voice at the other end. She had made this phone call five times prior to this—after four IUIs and one IVF.

She always said the same thing. 'You are not pregnant. You can stop the medicines. Come and meet Dr Leela once you get your period.'

This would be my cue to slump down and succumb to the mind-numbing sadness. But this time, as I waited for the well-rehearsed lines, Dr Preetha broke away from the script.

She said, 'You *are* pregnant. Your beta hCG value is 75. Come to the IVF clinic as soon as you can.'

After lunch I had a thirty-minute one-on-one meeting with the head of communications to understand his views on field documentation. I carried a portable voice recorder because I could not hear a single word anyone was saying. I then drove to the IVF clinic fifteen kilometres away, but I was as good as blindfolded because no piece of visual information pierced my senses. When I sat at Dr Preetha's desk, she dished out all the advice that is typically given to pregnant women. 'Eat healthy. Listen to music. Think positive. Whatever you do has an impact on your baby.' I turned once or twice to check if she was addressing someone else standing behind me. Me *pregnant*? My *baby*? This was an out-of-body experience.

As someone who had spent an inordinate amount of time, effort and financial resources on getting pregnant, I felt I knew more about reproductive medicine than practising medical professionals. And yet, because I had failed at it so many times, I no longer believed that ART would deliver the goods. It had become an unrealistic goal and I persevered only out of a sense of self-obligation. I owed it to myself and to Ranjith to try again and again, yet never truly believed that we would succeed. Therefore I, a veteran with years of training, was fully equipped to handle failure, but success left me completely baffled. For once, all my calculations about fertilization, implantation, beta hCG and HPTs had gone horribly wrong, and still everything had turned out terribly right. I *was* pregnant.

At some point during the discussion, after she had persuaded me into believing that I was *really* pregnant, Dr Preetha raised a couple of red flags.

'Your beta hCG levels are on the lower side and this indicates a possible risk of miscarriage. It could also be just a case of late implantation.'

'OK.'

'The presence of beta hCG by itself is not enough to confirm a healthy pregnancy. The value has to double in the next forty-eight hours. So day after tomorrow we will repeat the test to see if it is doubling. Only then can we be sure you are on track.'

'OK. Fine.'

I sat facing her, hands on the table, leaning forward to grasp every single word she was saying. Entrusted with an unexpected reward and responsibility, I wanted to make sure I understood all the variables and complexities.

'Is there anything *I* can do to help the pregnancy?'

She said the same things.

'Eat healthy. Listen to music. Think positive.'

~

Back in the car, I made the call to Ranjith that I had mimed and enacted countless times in the years that had gone by. He was excited and happy but not surprised. For me, the news of the pregnancy was like being hit by a meteorite from outer space, while for Ranjith it was as if he had been calculating this particular meteorite's trajectory all along and knew the precise point at which it would hit the earth's surface.

'Super kuttu!' he said again and again, as if this was my sole achievement. We smiled and laughed, having tasted the sweetness of success for the very first time. I did warn him about the risk of miscarriage, but he brushed it aside.

'I don't care. I know this will go through. And you and the baby will have the same birthday month. We are going to have an October baby.' His confidence was unshakeable, making me at once both happy and a little afraid.

Next in the hierarchy of information sharing was Amma. She was away in Lucknow attending a seminar. She hurriedly acknowledged what she heard but did not say anything more because she was in the midst of a session. Amma knew all about the cycles; the dates and outcomes of the IUIs, egg pick-ups, embryo transfers and beta hCG tests. She was a scientist herself and understood the chemical and biological processes underpinning fertility treatment. She had all the facts and data but *none* of the emotional subtext. We never talked about what I was going through internally. If she attempted to probe I would bring the shutters down on that conversation. She was supportive in the way all mothers are—worried about their children and wanting the best for them. But I was scared to open up about my inner chaos because I suspected it would end up upsetting *her* more than me. She was the brand ambassador for sentimentalism and melodrama, her face crumpling and dissolving into tears at the slightest provocation. I had to keep reminding her to be more matter-of-fact; *I had my own outbursts to deal with.* It was easier to discuss infertility with outsiders—those who were not invested in the result.

I shared the news with a couple of my friends from the office. Arun came to know because he was around when the call came. I blurted it out, unable to contain my disbelieving excitement. Of course, he had no clue about the IVF. Meera, on the other hand, was my IVF confidante. She was one of the first friends I made at the NGO and the first person I came out to about my struggles to conceive. Meera revealed that she too was starting out on the same path. I kept her updated about the daily highs and lows of the cycle. We would sneak in discussion about IVF during coffee breaks when others were not around. Her empathetic ears brought respite to my overworked IVF brain. She hugged and kissed me the next day when I told her, as if we had found success on a joint adventure.

Apart from these four, no one else knew. My in-laws were vaguely aware that some treatment was underway, but they were ignorant about the specifics. Ranjith and I did not volunteer information and they did not seek any either.

They were content to know that we were going to the doctors and doing *something* to have a baby. Ranjith's sister and my brother remained completely out of the loop. I was not intimate with Ranjith's sister, so that part was understandable, but my brother and I were thick as thieves. I didn't talk to Gopal about infertility because it was embarrassing. How can a sister discuss with her brother her bedroom challenges? Even if I could bring myself to talk to him about it, I didn't want him to share it with his wife Archana. It hurt my ego too much to let her have knowledge of my failings. Thus, we shared everything else, but sidestepped the active volcano simmering right in the middle of our lives.

For the most part Ranjith and I behaved like espionage agents executing a top-secret undercover operation. The world would find out when the mission was accomplished, but what went into pulling it off would remain forever classified. The secrecy was, however, a double-edged sword. It offered protection from prying and requests for updates, but it also meant we were denied the concern, sympathy and encouragement of our well-wishers. Even on the worst days of the month we could not afford to drop the guise of usualness.

~

Two days later I got another call from the clinic. It was Sini's voice at the other end. 'You owe us a treat,' she began.

The value of beta hCG was 150 mIU/ml. It had doubled exactly. The first ultrasound was scheduled for two weeks later. Again, I joyously informed the circle of people who were in the know about my pregnancy and began to count every minute of the lengthiest fortnight that had to pass before I could hear the baby's heartbeat.

At work I was in charge of organizing a workshop on documentation for colleagues from various parts of the country the following week. My heart was not in it; my heart was in staying at home and daydreaming about my baby and impending motherhood. My heart was in exercising utmost care and precaution in preserving this fledgling that had found shelter in my womb. But there was no way I could miss a workshop that *I* was organizing. It was unfair to foist it on another team member at the last minute, so I decided that I would continue with my work. Besides, this IVF cycle had been a charming tale of unexpected twists and turns so far. Every time I felt it was doomed, it resurrected itself back into reckoning. The low beta hCG values hung ominously in the air, signalling the danger of miscarriage, but I chose to ignore the blare of that siren. I was gazing at a blue-skied, sunshine-filled, butterfly-themed happily-ever-after.

I would be pregnant two more times after this, but I would never again feel the same gush of love and warmth as I did now. I was giddy as a teenager living her first crush. If someone said, 'Hello, how are you?', it took all my self-control to stop myself from saying, 'I am pregnant. Thank you.' *What else?* I walked with a spring in my step and a permanent grin on my face. From keeper of the disgraceful secret of infertility, I moved up to become keeper of the delightful secret of pregnancy, a secret I was confident the world would be envious of when it found out in due course. For now I carried it safely in my heart and womb, every now and then mentally retreating from the outside world to check on it. I cradled and nurtured my tiny seed of joy and mystery; it was my mission to protect its very existence. And thus, all my current and former loves from thirty-odd years of living were upstaged overnight and single-handedly by the baby.

11

Nothing Chemical about It

In what must have been my most disengaged week at work (and there have been many), I forced myself to sit through the sessions of the documentation workshop. Except, it was not enough for me to sit through it, I had to run it. This meant coordinating with participants and facilitators, ensuring sessions did not overrun, addressing logistical issues, from a dysfunctional projector to delayed lunch. This couldn't be done sitting in a corner with a laptop. I wanted to prioritize this pregnancy and restrain from too much physical or mental exertion. I wanted to walk slowly, avoid the stairs, drink less coffee and not get too stressed about anything. But this particular week could not accommodate any slowing down.

Anyway, I was not fully seduced by the idea that excess physical or mental activity could harm the baby. Everything I had read suggested that you could continue your regular routine while pregnant. So I tried to strike a balance between being cautious and at the same time carefree.

The workshop was taking place in a room on the seventh floor. The pantry was located on the fourth floor. So every tea and coffee break meant descending three levels. First, I would wait for the elevator. After precisely thirty seconds I would give up and walk towards the fire exit.

Floor VII to VI: Skip down the steps rapidly.

Floor VI: I am pregnant. I should cut down my pace.

Floor VI to V: Glide gently down the stairway.

Floor V: Does it really make a difference? Back to skipping.

Floor V to IV: But I must take every precaution since so little is in my hands. Back to gliding.

Floor IV to III: If this is a viable pregnancy, it will continue no matter how quickly I climb up and down the stairs, and if it is not, then the matter of how slowly I descend the stairs will be of no consequence. Back to skipping.

Floor III: Oh shoot! What am I doing on the third floor? Where's the elevator?

And thus I oscillated between a 'whatever-has-to-happen-will-happen' fatalism and a 'I-don't-want-to-take-a-step-wrong' kind of vigilance. Melting one moment, freezing another, my life as a nebulous cube of ice continued all week, until Friday arrived to put me out of my misery. In the evening I plopped myself on the rattan diwan at home and exhaled. Now I could focus on my baby.

Ranjith's parents visited us over the weekend. Achan (I call Ranjith's parents also Achan and Amma) retired as head of the R&D division of a public service undertaking situated on the outskirts of Bangalore. He had spent all his career with the same company, moving from one staff quarter to another in the same township. He took voluntary retirement before we got married and moved back to Ottappalam in Kerala. Even though his engineering talent had taken him around the world, from Japan to Germany to the US, he remained inside and outside a man rooted in his village, indifferent to cities and the changing times. In that way he was just like his wife, who steadfastly refused to have anything to do with the outside world. Amma was a devoted mother and wife who was content running her kitchen, tending to every flower and weed in her garden and supplicating the gods in the next-door temple with offerings for her children's well-being. Both Achan and Amma felt a strong affiliation with Bangalore, having spent over twenty-five years in its vicinity. They spoke Kannada fluently, relished bisi bele bhath and other Karnataka specials, and bought into the local customs. This and the love for their children ensured their monthly visits to Bangalore, shuttling between Ranjith's and their daughter Remya's homes.

They did not know about my pregnancy. We had decided to wait for the first ultrasound before announcing it to the family. But in the afternoon, when it was just Amma and me in the kitchen and she was updating me about all the weddings, births and deaths in the family, I felt it fit to announce my own contribution. I told her that I was pregnant. In fact, I had been bursting to tell her from the moment I found out.

By now we had already been married for more than six years, so when I told her I was pregnant I expected her to throw her hands in the air and scream, 'Finally!' All right, it was not that, but I anticipated *some* excitement, *some* emotion. Her response was totally unforeseen. She smiled benignly.

I thought she had not heard me correctly and I repeated myself.

Still nothing. This time she added, 'I will pray for you.'

I looked around to see if I was the only one who found this peculiar, but there was no one else around.

I carried on.

'I don't have any symptoms so far. No nausea, nothing...'

'*Aano*? That's strange. All of us had terrible nausea each time. You remember how Remya used to vomit after breakfast every day.'

'Hmm,' I smiled weakly.

So, I was the only weird one. I changed the topic abruptly. I had enough pre-existing tension about my not having any symptoms and put down her muted reaction to 'different people operate in different ways'. But inside I was crestfallen because I had rehearsed this scene in my head so many times. I knew how much Ranjith's parents adored children and how much they wanted to see both of us have a baby. My inability to conceive all these years had probably hit *them* the hardest outside us. Ranjith and I felt a sense of shame at being unable to fulfil this basic obligation that Indian children feel they owe their parents. I thought I was going to make them wildly happy by giving them this news but had clearly read them wrong. They were happy, but they were not the kind to make a fuss about it. They were happy, but guardedly so. They were happy, but nothing changed in their demeanour that day. There was not a single extra word or sentence from them on this topic.

In the evening Ranjith's sister brought her two-year-old and six-year-old to meet their grandparents. As in most families, all talk centred on the children. In the middle of tea and chatter, I felt a strong cramping in my abdomen. By now I was used to taking a bathroom break every twenty minutes to make an inspection, knowing that any sign of blood was bad news. So *any* twinge, prick or tug made me dart inside to check for spotting. So far every visit had proved to be unnecessary. This time, surrounded by all things pleasant and merry, I hesitated. Placing a hand protectively over my stomach, I stayed put.

The evening sky began to change colour and Achan insisted that Remya turn back. They had a long drive ahead of them. They said their goodbyes and left while I cleared the dishes, plumped up the cushions and brought the furniture back into alignment. It was also time for a postponed pee break. I had forgotten all about the cramping and my fingers undid the knot of the pyjama in habitual disregard. I sat on the commode holding up the lowered salwar when my eyes fell on my panties. I froze. There was blood. Dark red blood. The one thing that I never wanted to see had materialized and was staring me in the face.

The first thought that rushed to my brain was that this pregnancy is over. But I continued to sit on the commode and eye the thinly splashed, almost-brown blood for a long time, hoping I could make it vanish with my piercing gaze, hoping that if I looked long and hard enough it would cease to exist. Eventually I got up and left. Then I pulled Ranjith into our bedroom and latched the door.

We decided to call Dr Leela right away. She asked me to take bed rest and come to the hospital the next day for an ultrasound. I immediately lay down on my back, arms stretched and pinned to my sides like a corpse, scared to stir anything neck downwards. Ranjith sat with me on the bed googling causes of pregnancy-related bleeding on his laptop.

He read out from websites what I already knew. A significant percentage of women experience some kind of bleeding during pregnancy. Caused by implantation or cervical changes, it is usually not a threat to the foetus, nor does it come in the way of full-term healthy babies. So, bleeding did not necessarily equate with a failing pregnancy. In the last two weeks I had agonized over the absence of any 'pregnancy symptoms'—nausea, fatigue, sore breasts. I hoped the bleeding was a 'pregnancy symptom', since some spotting was expected in every pregnancy. Maybe *this* was the surest sign so far of my pregnant status. *You see my desperation, don't you?*

I spent the whole night in a frigid, motionless state, only getting up for bathroom breaks. Fortunately, there were no more bouts of bleeding. Sleep came intermittently, and there was a lengthy, bizarre dream in which I went for the ultrasound to find my foetus was already at full term and I was sent in for labour. When I opened my eyes the next morning I recounted the dream to Ranjith. Both of us understood it to mean that this pregnancy would reach its logical end. We interpreted it as auguring a positive outcome. While getting dressed to leave for the hospital, I felt almost grateful that the ultrasound had been brought forward. My date with the baby had been advanced.

It was a Sunday and the IVF clinic did not open on Sundays, so we had to go to the main hospital to which the clinic was attached for the ultrasound. The IVF clinic was my comfort zone. I knew its residents and rhythms, and they knew me. I didn't have to rehash history or explain the stakes linked to a test or procedure. They knew an ultrasound was not just an ultrasound; it was the culmination of years of desire and heartbreak. But in the large, impersonal environs of a multi-speciality hospital, an ultrasound was just another set of black-and-white images on a computer screen. And, outside the IVF ecosystem, even medical professionals knew very little about infertility treatment or the sensitivity required in communicating with those at the receiving end.

First, we had a difficult time convincing the nurse at radiology to schedule an ultrasound. She asked us to wait until Monday and get the doctor to prepone the ultrasound prescription, since on paper it was not meant to be done until a week later. I only had a verbal instruction from Dr Leela on the phone to get it done immediately. To the nurse it seemed absurd that I was insisting on an ultrasound on a Sunday when I did not have the correct date on the prescription and it was clearly not an emergency. I stood my ground. She then tried to dissuade me by saying that only male technicians were available. I said I didn't care. Then she asked me to fill my bladder. I told her that this had to be a trans-vaginal ultrasound and we needed an empty bladder. I was only six weeks pregnant and an abdominal ultrasound would not be useful at this point. By now I was beginning to get concerned about the overall competence of the radiology department. Even if they inserted their magic wand into my vagina, would they know what to look for?

Finally, I was undressed and a radiologist stepped in to do the needful. He seemed mild-mannered and conscientious. He was respectful of my nudity, averting his gaze while inserting the probe inside. He spent almost fifteen minutes scouring the insides of my uterus for any signs of a live foetus. I kept my eyes fixed on his face for the slightest clue that it might give me about my fate. At the end of the session he said, 'You are not pregnant.' There was only a large cyst in my uterus, no gestational sac, no foetus.

He didn't say that I had miscarried. He said that I was *not* pregnant, *had never been.*

I insisted, 'No. Look at my beta hCG results. I *am* pregnant.' I was not going to give up my hard-earned, hard-fought pregnancy so easily.

He shrugged his shoulders.

I tried again, 'This is an IVF pregnancy. I got a positive pregnancy test a week ago. I am sure I am pregnant.'

He just stared blankly at me. He hadn't heard of the beta hCG test and was not about to take medical lessons from a patient. In his view I was delusional. What I needed was psychiatric evaluation, not a pregnancy.

How much more could I argue medicine with a licenced doctor? I gave up the fight, got dressed and walked out of the hospital with the report of the ultrasound in hand. We would have to wait until Monday to know where this pregnancy stood.

As Ranjith and I crossed the IVF clinic on our way out, we decided to test our rotten luck further and check if anyone was inside. On some Sundays the clinic would be open for a few hours to accommodate an ovum pick-up or an embryo transfer. In what turned out to be the only piece of good fortune of the previous twenty-four hours, the clinic was open and Sini was around. Seeing her was like finding the mother ship when hit by an iceberg; here was someone who would take me under her wings, who *knew* I was pregnant. Someone who wouldn't annul my pregnancy on a technicality.

I quickly explained the bleeding episode and shoved the dossier of images into her hands urging her to find my missing foetus. She took a minute to study the ultrasound report and confirmed what I already suspected. This was most likely a chemical pregnancy.

A chemical pregnancy is a loss which takes place *after* the pregnancy test but *before* the ultrasound. The slip between the cup and the lip. This meant that the embryo had implanted in my uterus and had started producing the hCG hormone, which was detected by the pregnancy test. But sometime after the positive result, the embryo failed to grow any further and my body decided to abort the foetus. Sini rang up Dr Leela from the clinic and informed her. The doctor ordered another beta hCG test. By now, in a healthy pregnancy, the beta hCG levels would have been in the range of thousands. If a fresh beta hCG test showed that the levels of the hormone had not spiked the way they were supposed to or were falling, we could safely conclude that this was going south. The outcome was obvious, but we still had to follow through with the protocol step by step before arriving at that conclusion.

I hated the label taped to my pregnancy. There was something so cruel about the term 'chemical pregnancy'. It seemed to suggest that a 'chemical pregnancy' was not a 'real' pregnancy. No real blood or tissue was involved, just a laboratory experiment gone awry, a few ounces of hormones gone astray. It was a term that stripped gestation of all its warmth and glow, discrediting what it sought to describe. Chemical pregnancy, by definition, suggested not a 'biological' pregnancy, and if you extended that line of reasoning, then the loss of a 'fake' pregnancy was not to be taken seriously either.

I refused to buy the term. It was an affront to my pride to get pregnant after all these years and then be stuck with a pitiless label. I would not allow it to undermine the dignity of what I had gained and lost. However early the loss may have been, my pregnancy was real and precious. I felt like I had lost a whole child, a child I had just begun to love and care for, a child I had promised to bring into this world and guard with all my strength. This loss was the death of that promise, and calling it a chemical pregnancy or some such technicality was going to be no shield against the pain.

I did not want to go home and face my in-laws, so we drove around town aimlessly. Then we stopped at a posh seafood restaurant and had a lavish lunch. I may have cried a few errant tears in between and Ranjith may have looked at me helplessly, wondering when this was going to end. It was almost evening by the time we returned home. I went about busily tidying up the house, which had been left in disarray in the morning's hurry to reach the hospital, careful to avoid any eye contact with my in-laws.

Ranjith's parents were as solemn to the loss as they had been to the news that I was pregnant. Achan did ask me if I could take some medicine or treatment to reverse the miscarriage. I did not expect him to spend all his waking hours reading up on reproductive medicine like I did, but even by layperson standards this sounded absurd. No, it is not possible to revive a lost pregnancy. If it was, wouldn't we just get down to doing it? I knew he was coming from a place of concern and that he and Amma were pained by the news, but on the surface it seemed as if they hadn't grasped its gravity. Just because I never revealed my wounds it did not mean I was not bleeding.

This reflected our overall relationship, which was built on the 'arm's length' principle. Our conversations were mostly transactional. Has the maid come? Is Ranjith travelling? What's for dinner? We guarded our territories and kept our secrets, careful not to cross boundaries. There was no outright conflict or animosity. It was always pleasant and cordial, but at the end of the day we were like strangers who had met on a long-distance train journey and didn't know what to do once the pleasantries were over. The forced proximity was awkward after a point, and we wished to retreat to our own devices. Yet, at a time of grief and vulnerability, I wished we were not so distant. Perhaps they did not know what to say. That is true of a lot of people when confronted by tragic circumstances such as illness or death. Perhaps they had no understanding of infertility science and did not know what to make of a pregnancy that folded up so early. Perhaps they felt it was best not to talk about the loss in case it upset me further. I don't know. I only wish we were not so cut off in our individual silos of pain.

12

Calling

I grew up thinking my life was very 'ordinary'. Middle-class family—check. Average looks—check. Average intelligence—check. Dull personality—check. Nothing exceptional ever happened to me. Life followed a steady course—school, college, job. Check. Check. Check—no great twists and turns, a nondescript existence.

But in my secret imagination I craved fame and glory, a world of public acclaim and recognition. There had to be a calling to my life, a higher purpose. What was my special mission to accomplish? What were my special skills or abilities or talents? To start a company? Become a poet? Champion a social cause? At twenty-two, as I exited the portals of the institute in Hyderabad, I was vexed by the need to find my calling. As soon as I apprehended it, I knew I would transform into the changing-the-face-of-the-world type of icon that I was always meant to be.

At first I believed it was my duty to carry on the family vocation. My mother is a teacher; my grandmother was one. As if in preparation, while in primary school, I would routinely line up pillows on the bed, wave a ruler at them and write indecipherable lessons on the doors of our bedroom cupboards with a piece of chalk pilfered from school. Everyone could see I was a natural. When I joined college, the time had come to put my skills to the test on the ground. I started offering tuition in French to a neighbour's schoolgoing daughter. My miserable Hindi had forced me to drop the subject after school and take up what seemed like a relatively easier second-language option in college. We would meet for an hour three days a week after college. But the fallacy that I had been nurturing since childhood soon came crashing down. It was one thing to lecture mute pillows and another to lock eyes and horns with a yawning thirteen-year-old. She had little interest in the subject of study and I did not have the teaching talent to make it come alive. I began hoping that my student wouldn't turn up for class. Even on the days she did turn up, my zeal to tutor her was even less than hers to be tutored. Only the one thousand rupees I received at the end of the month from her mother kept me going. No, teaching was not my calling.

I graduated from the institute in Hyderabad in 2004. I had no intention of going back to Trivandrum and started looking for jobs in the city. A good majority of those who came to the institute intended to do an MPhil or a PhD and finish up at some university, combining research with teaching. By the final year, a few of my peers were already writing the Graduate Record Examinations (GRE) and leafing through the prospectuses of American schools. Some of my friends did look for jobs, but maximum approval was reserved for those who wished to pursue higher studies. I figured that I had to go to the US and do a PhD. That was the minimum level of educational qualification I expected of myself. Besides, my mother had a PhD in biochemistry. *How could I fall short of that standard?*

I looked up to my mother in more ways than I admitted. She had emphasized throughout my childhood the importance of a career. She herself was fiercely invested in her teaching job—publishing papers in journals, travelling to seminars and conferences, mentoring dozens of PhD scholars. She wrote her PhD thesis while pregnant with her first child and went back to work two months after I was born, leaving me in the care of grandparents. She told me repeatedly to build my own professional path and not be dependent on husband or family for my fulfilment. I grew up subconsciously imbibing these lessons. Even later, work was my asylum. Through all the highs and lows of fertility treatment my work offered a sense of continuity and progress. Every time a cycle of treatment failed, I went back to it with double the attention and interest. I told myself, 'Thank God I have my job to return to.'

~

At the end of the MA programme, Amma and Achan made it clear that they could not finance my educational aspirations any further. They didn't see any value in my securing a doctorate from a foreign university when the same degree was available locally and at one-tenth of the cost. So the only option left for me was to find a job that would allow me to do so.

An English daily was looking for reporters and was open to hiring candidates without a journalism background. After a brief interview I joined the team of reporters and editors that managed the lifestyle pages at ten thousand rupees per month plus extra for bylines. Two days after my course wound up,

I started the job. Since I had no place to stay, I continued in the institute hostel, which was desolate by then, the residents having left for the summer break.

That job was the perfect mismatch between abilities and requirement, between work and worker. It was my responsibility to put together the high-profile opening page of the Friday supplement. Later, I learnt that the other team members were surprised that a newbie had been assigned this 'crown jewel'. The page was designed to have a lead article and one or two smaller write-ups. A day before the supplement was meant to go to press, the marketing team would inform us about the space left for content after the placing of advertisements. On a good day I needed only one lead article; the rest of the page would be taken up by advertisements for apparel, jewellery or weekend entertainment. On bad days I needed all three. Since this was the opening page, it had to be flashy, attention-grabbing, and pegged to celebrity lives. But I found myself totally unworthy of the flagship page. I was a bumbling, fumbling, nervous wreck of a journalist who was always short of story ideas, who could not write catchy headlines or pick sexy photos from the image library, and who struggled to suture celebrities into every write-up. I did not have the outgoing and intrepid personality, the mental agility or even the street-smarts that a reporter needs. After every weekly editorial meeting I felt so inept that I wanted to pick up my handbag and scoot from the building and job, eager to put a quick end to the misery of my paltry journalistic skills.

On my day off I would ring up Gopal and have hour-long conversations about the unsuitability of my job. He was wise beyond his years and urged me to persevere. Amma and Achan also said the same things: 'Every job has its advantages and disadvantages; no job is perfect. Hang in there for a year and things will get easier.'

Well, things did begin to look up after a couple of months, and the event responsible for the change in tide was an interview with the writer Amitav Ghosh. This assignment allowed me to put to use my background in English literature. I had read Ghosh's novels, and familiarity with Indian writing in English enabled me to jot down some half-intelligent questions prior to the meeting. I met Amitav Ghosh in the lobby of a five-star hotel, where he was having a series of press interactions to promote his new novel. He got up to shake hands with me and we sat down in a secluded corner for the interview. He was gentle, thoughtful and modest to a fault, responding at length to my questions while I scribbled down his responses furiously on a notepad balanced on my lap. The thirty-minute interview went smoothly, and at the end Amitav Ghosh himself appeared pleased. A few copies of his new book, *The Hungry Tide*, were arranged in a spiral on the coffee table. He picked one up, asked my name again and wrote an inscription before handing it over. I blushed and said 'Thank you' a few dozen times before being escorted outside. Later, Ghosh remarked to his publisher, who passed on the information to my editor, that *this* girl was the 'best of the lot'.

News of Ghosh's praise spread like wildfire in the newsroom. My prestige shot up and the chief editor herself called me into her room and said teasingly, 'How does it feel to floor Amitav Ghosh?' Needless to say, Ghosh became my favourite author. I pledged to read every book he ever wrote and floated in the stratosphere dreaming of all the literary giants I was going to floor in the future. I didn't have to wait very long. The next Indian writer in English was waiting just around the corner.

A month later, Hyderabad was getting ready to host a literary conference, and no prizes for guessing who was designated to cover it. The biggest literary name attending that event was Vikram Seth. My first task was to get an interview with the man. I went to the airport to receive him along with other members of the organizing committee. I almost missed recognizing the writer in the airport melee. He came with no celebrity airs or entourage. He wore a kurta, picked a gigantic suitcase off the carousel, the strain of the effort visible on his face, and walked to the exit gate. Once the organizers had finished their introductions, I stepped up and requested him for an interview. He said 'yes', but I would have to meet him at his hotel room in thirty minutes. I ran out, flagged down an auto and bid the driver to fly to the hotel. On the way I rang up our photographer and asked him to race to the hotel too.

Seth invited me to his room. We had only fifteen minutes before he had to rush out for a banquet dinner downstairs. I sat on the sofa with the same notepad on my lap and began with some stock generic questions jotted in the auto ride on the way to the hotel. 'How does it feel to be in Hyderabad?' 'What do you enjoy writing more—poetry or prose?' 'Your thoughts on the conference?' I had not done my research on Seth and was trying and failing simultaneously at winging it. The embarrassing truth was that I had not expected him to agree to an interview right away. My plan was to ask for some time, but he asked to meet immediately. How could I refuse? I was trapped. He was down to earth and courteous, even going so far as to show interest in my background, but I had nothing noteworthy to say or ask.

During the course of the conversation, I did notice that he seemed very pale and troubled. I assumed he was exhausted from the journey. But Seth revealed that his mama had just passed away. *What? His mother had just died.* He was very close to his mama and had been in two minds about making this trip, but only came this far because he did not want to renege on a prior commitment. I expressed my condolences and wound up the interview as abruptly and sketchily as it had begun.

Back at the newsroom I told everyone that Vikram Seth's mother had just passed away. Leila Seth, the first woman to be the chief justice of a state high court, was a noted figure in her own right, and this was breaking news. The news team began checking their sources for further details, while the features team was baffled that he had chosen to leave his mother's funeral and attend a literary event. The news team was not able to verify the information and decided not to carry it despite my insistence that I had it from the horse's mouth. I wrote my piece on Seth and went home.

While eating dinner in the hostel canteen, the events of the day were flashing in my head in playback mode. It did seem odd that Seth had chosen to come to Hyderabad after having suffered such an immense bereavement. Something was not sitting right. Had I not heard him correctly? Had I misunderstood him? And then I broke into a cold sweat.

He meant 'maama', the Hindi 'maama', meaning uncle, perhaps his mother's brother. His clipped British accent had thrown me off, and I had confused 'maama' with 'mama', meaning mother. And I thought I had a scoop! If only I had kept it to myself! Now I had to clarify this to the entire newsroom. What if they had taken me at my word and published this? How could I have saved face? I was ready to bury myself where I sat from my mortification at the thought. *Why hadn't I scooted earlier?*

Before I could do worse and sink the newspaper itself, good sense prevailed and I resigned from my position. No, newspaper reporting was not my calling.

Next up, book publishing. Interacting with the editor who escorted Amitav Ghosh made me wonder if I should explore prospects in the world of books and writers. A professor from the institute put me in touch with a publishing house that specialized in textbooks for schools and colleges. They asked me to take up an assignment on a freelance basis to test my skills and aptitude. I completed the assignment, they offered me a job and I was back in action.

This time I moved into a paying guest facility, sharing a room with two others in the sixth-floor apartment of a building in the centre of town. The flat was spacious and had four bedrooms, shared by fifteen girls who came and left at different times of the day, rarely all present at the same time. Of the fifteen girls, fourteen worked in either Satyam or Infosys. When I said I worked for a publishing house, they appeared puzzled. 'Hardware?' They asked. *If it was not software, what else could it be?*

Publishing was sedate. There was none of the adventure or glamour of media and none of the stress and panic either. A book took months to publish; there were no daily deadlines. There were only four copy editors in the company and we became a close set. And thus began a phase of my life that I value the most—living all alone in a big, strange city, solely responsible for my safety, finances and entertainment, unprotected by the safety net of parents, local guardians, connections, or even a proper home. There are few things as thrilling and as lonely in this world. On some days it was like being in a spinning ferris wheel at its peak, surveying a miniature landscape from my vantage point, intoxicated by the potent drugs of youth and freedom. On other days it was humbling to be brought down to earth by the knowledge of my own smallness and aloneness in a vast, uncaring city.

At this point I still entertained ideas of working for a year, saving enough money to appear for GRE and then applying to a university in the US for a PhD programme. Every now and then I would hear of a classmate who was flying off to NYU or Berkeley and would feel the pang of unfinished business. So six months after joining the publishing house I signed up for GRE coaching classes. In all earnest I woke up at the crack of dawn, hailed an autorickshaw to the coaching centre, sat bleary-eyed through English and maths lessons, and when done, hailed another autorickshaw to reach office by nine. But, as is usually the case when you join an after-hours class, the whole universe conspires to make it impossible to attend.

Around the same time, our publishing house went into a frenzy over a new textbook due for release in a couple of months. It had to be written, edited *and* published in two months. It was an impossible deadline. The book had been commissioned by the government and was expected to sell thousands of copies. It was a high-stakes contract to win and we couldn't afford to miss the delivery date; the academic year had already begun and pupils were waiting for the textbook. All the editors were asked to drop other manuscripts and pool their combined strength to see this through. This meant long hours in office, surrendering weekends, breathing down the typesetters' necks to design pages and make copy-editing changes. I didn't make it beyond the first week of GRE coaching.

After the book fever subsided and we went back to saner rhythms, I picked up the scattered bits of my PhD dream, pondering what needed to be done. By now the shine of a doctorate degree and life abroad had started to fade. Life in Hyderabad was quite appealing. I had a comfortable job, financial independence and personal freedom. Did I really wish to forsake all that and travel to a foreign country to live in a university dorm for four years? Was it worth the shake-up? Maybe not. But I felt that a PhD *per se* was unavoidable. Academic publishing houses look for highly educated editors with deep subject knowledge—for instance, a science doctorate for a science editor. The others in the editorial team either had a PhD or were on their way to getting one. A PhD was inevitable; the only question open to debate was where to get one.

Amending my plans, I started scouting for universities in south India. There was a centre in Bangalore that offered doctoral programmes in culture studies. I attached my CV, a writing sample and the thesis proposal, and sent in the application. My proposed subject was television soap operas in Kerala, particularly *Stree*, a pioneer in mega-serials centred on an iconic female character who was self-sacrificing, chaste and obedient. The subject complemented my interest in media and gender studies, and if selected would give me the advantage of spending time in Trivandrum under the guise of data collection. Soon enough, I was called for an interview to Bangalore. There weren't many seats available, but I felt reasonably confident of getting one.

That day was something of a perfect storm. First, my train arrived late. I was staying at a friend's house and had to speed up bath and breakfast to reach the centre. I did call the interview coordinator and inform her about the delayed train, but it made me feel off-balance even before reaching the venue. Once I entered the building and absorbed its atmosphere, the other candidates and their conversations, I felt even more deflated. Many of them had already completed an MPhil and therefore had additional preparation for a PhD. They knew their Derrida and Foucault, postmodernism and postcolonialism, cultural hegemony and identity politics, while my critique of mega-serials was beginning to look too plain and shallow. The two years of working had widened the schism between me and academics.

That interview did not last very long. There were three panellists and two questions.

Right off the bat, one of the interviewers, a bespectacled senior gentleman, said, 'There is nothing new in this proposal. There are tonnes of feminist critiques of mega soaps. Is there anything *more* you want to add which hasn't been covered here?'

He held my one-and-a-half-page write-up with such disdain that I found myself dissolving into the revolving chair.

'Hmm . . . no,' I admitted. I had spent a month and all my intellectual capital drafting this. If there was something *more* to add, why would have I waited for him to ask? Besides, I was caught off guard by his bluntness. He didn't waste even a couple of minutes on 'So, tell us about your proposal' before sharing this feedback.

After a pause, he said, 'OK. Do you have any questions for us then?' He seemed grateful that I was at least honest about my intellectual bankruptcy, not wasting any more of their time.

'Hmm . . . no,' I admitted again, having gone blank by then.

Unfortunately, I had started drinking the coffee and nibbling the biscuit that was placed in front of me and was left to contend with two minutes of awkward silence while I finished both, tucked my tail in and scurried out on the first bus back to Hyderabad. I didn't even wait for the list of selected candidates to be announced.

I have never felt so talentless in my life as I did then. On the journey back I thanked the one million gods in the Hindu pantheon for my job. I still had that to return to. No, a PhD was not my calling.

After that, I continued with editing, writing, and grappling with content. It was the least disastrous of all my professional escapades. Can it be described as a 'calling'? Maybe not. It's more likely a preference. I don't think I *have* a calling, an unchanging, unflagging devotion to one idea, cause or line of work. Those who do, I envy, but I am not one of them. Wait. Does online shopping and arguing with customer support executives count?

13

Third Time's the Charm?

Soon after the ultrasound that confirmed the chemical pregnancy, I got my period, which lasted more than two weeks. The bleeding started, stopped, then restarted, in what seemed like an endless cycle. The blood went from red to brown to black, and slimy, amoeba-like clots squeezed themselves out. Along with the fluid and semi-solid matter, my ache and sense of betrayal too dribbled away, giving rise to a faint hope and consolation. At least I got pregnant this time. My uterus and ovaries, which had failed at conception despite years of pushes and shoves from medicine, had finally done something right. The reproductive engine had stuttered and sputtered and even rumbled some distance before dying down again. It made me believe that if it can happen once, it can happen again.

There were other rationales, too, for reassurance. To my absolute astonishment, I had watched myself fall in love with my unborn child. All the days of the fortnight that the pregnancy lasted I was carried by a wave of excitement and emotion. Until then I was so focused on the mechanics of reproduction that I had forgotten about its ultimate outcome—a classic case of not seeing the forest for the trees. But this short fling with motherhood left me awash with the heady rush and heartache of falling in love. It was a teaser for the sweetness of motherhood. I couldn't wait for the full-length affair.

The miscarriage also evened my karmic scores, I felt. Most infertility survivors have experienced a loss or two before going on to have a baby. I couldn't expect to be the exception to the rule. There was cosmic debt to clear in the form of failed attempts or miscarriages. This miscarriage was therefore the obligatory failure that would act as the precursor to success.

The biggest reason for hope lay in the five embryos left over from the previous cycle, which had been frozen and stored in the IVF laboratory. The surplus embryos are preserved at −196°C, and when they need to be transferred to a woman's body the frozen cells are thawed and allowed to grow in an IVF lab before being placed back in the uterus. A frozen embryo transfer (FET) is cheaper and easier when compared with a full-length IVF cycle. Since embryos have already been harvested, one can skip the first and more gruelling half of a fresh IVF cycle—stimulating the ovaries to produce eggs. However, freezing and thawing of embryos is a risky process. The cells are exposed to an extremely harsh and toxic environment and some embryos may fail to survive. There was a good chance that of the five embryos remaining, at least one or two would end up as collateral damage. I hoped I had enough for at least two more attempts.

Doctors advise a minimum gap of three to four months between two IVF cycles to allow the body time for restoration.

I waited, and about six months after the loss I was back at the IVF clinic in August 2013, emotionally and physically ready to try to become pregnant again. Once I finished consulting Dr Leela, I went back to the nurses' station to chat with Sini. I had noticed her stomach bulging through the blue uniform and wanted to confirm my suspicion.

We knew each other well enough for me to ask right away, 'Are you pregnant?'

She blushed, her heart-shaped face breaking into a wide grin.

'Yes.'

'Oh great! Why didn't you tell me? How far along are you?'

'Sorry. I found out soon after your last cycle. I thought I would message you once I finished the first trimester but then it slipped my mind. I am due in November.'

'That's fine. Congratulations! I am so happy for you,' I said, and held her hands, starting a twenty-minute conversation on whether it had happened naturally, how she found out, what her symptoms were . . . basically, gathering reference material to be banked for future use.

Only when I stepped into the elevator to go down to the parking lot did I switch off the smile and excitement. I felt truly happy for her, there was no deceit in that. But there was also the weight of a hundred bricks in my chest. Partly because *she* was pregnant and *I* was not. This jealousy and resentment reared its head every time someone I knew got pregnant. In Sini's case it was partly because I did not want to go through IVF without her. She was in the middle of her second trimester and would go on maternity leave in a couple of months. I wanted to get pregnant while she was still around.

Sini had been the nursing assistant for every single procedure of mine in the last two years. IVF cycles involve a lot of waiting, like any hospital visit, and I gravitated towards her during those intervals. While I rested in the recovery room after an IUI or an embryo transfer, she would keep me entertained. Inventorying instruments and medicines or giving instructions to housekeeping staff, she chatted about the day-to-day dilemmas and complications in her own life—how to buy a second-hand car online, hire a reliable house help or her own attempts to get pregnant. Typically, there weren't many other patients to care for, making it possible for the nurses to direct individual attention towards their patients. We stayed in touch even outside the IVF cycles, wishing each other on festival days and birthdays.

Over time, I have seen medical professionals become inured to suffering. They see so much of it every day. Whatever you have, they have seen much worse. But Sini's empathy was intact, uneroded by the daily demands on it. She offered to pray for me at her church every Sunday and celebrated my triumphs and bemoaned my disasters. The questions or concerns I was too intimidated to ask Dr Leela, Sini answered for me. Every time I walked into the clinic and saw her face, I reckoned I had reached someplace familiar; her face neutralized the cold, uninviting, antiseptic ambience of the clinic.

Losing such a valuable ally and placing myself in the hands of some unknown nurse to whom I was just another IVF patient was not a welcome proposition. I kept my fingers crossed. This was going to be IVF attempt number three. The first attempt did not result in a pregnancy. The second attempt resulted in a pregnancy that wrapped up in an early miscarriage. Was I going to be third-time lucky?

~

In an FET cycle, you have a head start. It is a relay race where the baton has now reached the last sprinter, who must build on the advantage and get to the finish line. There are some injections and ultrasounds as in a full-fledged IVF cycle, but because the embryos are already in cold storage there is no pressure on the uterus. The only expectation is a thickened endometrium. The endometrium, or the uterine lining, grows as the menstrual cycle progresses towards ovulation, allowing an embryo to implant itself easily. However, if implantation does not take place, it disintegrates, resulting in the bleeding that happens during a period. In an FET cycle, the embryo transfer is performed when the endometrium reaches an optimal level of thickness.

My endometrial lining reached a favourable thickness of 8.9 mm. Praveen picked three out of the five embryos for thawing. I had an odd number of embryos left, which meant they had to be transferred back in unequal combinations of three and two. Doctors prefer to place at least two embryos inside the uterus to improve the odds of achieving a pregnancy. All the embryos were frozen three days after fertilization; they were all grade-A and had reached the eight-cell stage, except for one. The last one was grade-B and had only six cells. It was decided that two grade-A eight-cell embryos and the iffy-looking grade-B six-cell embryo would be transferred into my uterus. I would still have two grade-A eight-cell embryos left for a final try.

This time Dr Leela advised forty-eight hours of bed rest after the transfer. In addition, I decided to work from home for the next two weeks until the beta hCG test. A mental autopsy of the last cycle led me to believe that the stress of commuting forty kilometres every day and the daily pressures of office life had played a part in sabotaging the pregnancy. Like every other woman fighting infertility, I blamed myself for each failure. *Perhaps driving had nothing to do with it, but it was still worthwhile to rule out that cause.* I got the necessary permission from my manager, informed colleagues and other associates that I would take all meetings on the phone for the next fifteen days, and converted our bedroom into my home office. And thus began my two-week wait until the beta hCG.

I was an old-timer at two-week waits, having endured them in multiple IUI and IVF cycles. But I never had to be at home during the entire period; going to work helped pause the infertility broadcast running inside my brain for at least a few hours in the day. Now there was all the time and space in the world to speculate endlessly about the verdict. Will the embryos implant? If they implant, will they develop further? What will be the value of hCG? If the value is high enough, will it double in the next forty-eight hours? And so on and so forth. It was going to be two interminably long weeks spent adding and subtracting, multiplying and dividing expectations from the cycle.

A woman who gets pregnant naturally has typically no idea what is going on inside her body until she misses her period. She wakes up one day, realizes her period is more than usually late and takes a pregnancy test. She probably has to endure two full minutes of not knowing before the

HPT displays the double pink line. I can't imagine the state of blissful ignorance, the serendipity, of just finding out one fine morning that you are pregnant. What a fine morning that would be (of course, assuming you wanted the pregnancy)! My life was the polar opposite of that scenario. I was tracking my embryos on a minute-by-minute, day-by-day basis in microscopic, cellular-level detail. I was pregnant even before I was pregnant and feared taking one breath wrong for the harm it might cause to my eight-cell wonders. I knew too much about the back end to be absolved of responsibility. It would have been a relief to restore reproductive illiteracy, at least temporarily. But since there was no erasing the knowledge that had been acquired incrementally and so painstakingly, I had to keep acquiring more and more of it to stay on top of the confusion and uncertainty. And, as with everything, the Internet was my number one accomplice. The Internet has been my friend, philosopher and guide in all of life's decision-making, but IVF made us inseparable. Daily, the questions in my head were unbundled and laid out at Google's feet.

I asked:

FET—pregnant?

FET after miscarriage—pregnant?

FET with 2 grade-A 8-cell embryos—pregnant?

No symptoms after FET with 2 grade-A 8-cell embryos—pregnant?

Just pregnant, anyone?

All my free time (maybe two to three hours on a working day) was spent on the laptop and smartphone, visiting websites, discussion boards, blog posts and support groups dedicated to infertility. In the process, I stumbled upon a whole new universe of meaning. An entire subculture existed on the Internet, created and owned by women who were fighting to get pregnant. It had its own code, lingo and dogma. Posts were peppered with acronyms.

DH = dear husband
TTC = trying to conceive
Aunt flo = period
1dp5dt = one day post-five-day embryo transfer
BFP = big fat positive
BFN = big fat negative

Subscribers put up their infertility history in their profile descriptions or signature lines, bypassing the need to keep recounting their painful record of past failings, letting people know where they stood at this point in their journey.

DH 32, Me 28
TTC Oct 2009,
4 IUIs, 2 IVFs
2 Miscarriages 2010—2012

Some profiles were intimidating. Seven IVFs, multiple back-to-back miscarriages, stillbirths. Such profiles commanded respect and authority in the forums. These profiles were of women who had been through every conceivable scenario and had inputs for every type of condition. I wondered if my own struggle would be so arduous. Would I end up as an infertility veteran?

It was my pastime to peruse profiles and count the number of attempts, the number of miscarriages or the number of years that it took women to achieve a BFP. Or I would check how many had got pregnant at the exact same stage I was in at the time. How many at IVF no. 1? Or how many at IVF no. 2 FET no. 1? I would use this data to arrive at an estimation of when I would be pregnant, corroborating my history with that of others. Who else was like me and had found success? Who was my IVF twin? But the Internet, as everyone knows, is a deep, dark well echoing your own voice. You only hear what you want to hear. I was an expert at tweaking reality to suit search results. If the two didn't match, then I was ready to hit results page twenty-one to find something that authenticated my beliefs.

There were subgroups dedicated to different procedures; there were IUI groups, IVF groups and surrogacy groups. I started actively stalking these forums only after my IVF cycles because I was very hopeful and confident during the IUI days, targeting a maximum time frame of three months to get pregnant. With every successive miss, the digging on the net got deeper. I did not post messages on any of the forums because it seemed as if everything had already been asked and answered. A simple Google search was enough to find multiple threads on the same topic. I felt shy and diffident in any social group, and even the anonymity of the Internet didn't make things easier. I was content to prowl in the background, listening to everyone without being heard. Discussions ranged from scientific queries and pleas to find out who else was in the same situation to requests to hear some positive stories.

The transfer was done a week ago; 2 grade-A blastocysts. The HPT today was negative. Is it too early? I feel I am pregnant. How long should I wait to repeat the HPT?

Is anyone doing an IVF this month or having an FET?

I am in the stimulation phase of my IVF cycle no 3. Feeling exceptionally low. I need to hear some success stories. Help!

Responses were mostly quick and everyone was forthcoming and empathetic. If you needed technical assistance, there was technical assistance. If you needed support, there was support. If you needed baby dust sent your way, baby dust was sent your way. Unified by unfortunate circumstances, this was a sisterhood in action. Most importantly, everyone wished success for the other. IVF is not a zero-sum game. The greater the number of us achieving pregnancy, the better the prognosis for everyone. Naturally, when someone else got a BFP while you got a BFN, it was sad, but it gave hope to the community at large. Maybe that month it was not your turn, but not too far in the future it would be yours.

~

The embryo transfer took place on a Thursday in August 2013. I stayed at home and took bed rest on Friday and Saturday, as indicated in the discharge summary. On Sunday, Ranjith had to travel to Mysore to attend to a farm he had bought in partnership with some school friends. He was going to return only in the evening. I was all alone at home, stuck inside on a purposeless, good-for-nothing Sunday morning. I had not brushed my teeth, taken a bath or made my bed. I ate bread and peanut butter for breakfast and planned to reheat leftovers from the previous night for lunch. After breakfast I went back to bed, my shabby self indistinguishable from the crumpled sheets. To bring some cheer to such a slow, bleak day, I speed-dialled my brother. Of course, Gopal didn't know that I had just completed an embryo transfer.

Gopal was the archetypal Malayalee son who had knocked off all the items on the parental checklist. He studied computer science engineering, secured campus placement in a software company, married at the age of twenty-eight a girl chosen by his mother and settled down to a life of south Indian domestic bliss in Chennai. In contrast, my score as a daughter was abysmal, I having failed at the least thing my family expected of me.

But he and I shared a warm and easy chemistry. We pulled each other's legs and understood each other's predicaments, even though a good part of our childhood was spent in trying to rip the other person's arm off its socket. Once we reached our late teens the fights paled. We had matured and mellowed down, and I realized that it was a no-contest. It was wiser to call for a truce with an opponent who stood six feet three inches tall, all bone and muscle. Then we became comrades, standing arm-in-arm against the common enemy, because few other adversities can bring you closer than a shared set of parents. We saw each other through Amma's bouts of shrill rants, Achan's morose silences, weddings of folks you had no idea were family, and visiting relatives who laid claim to your room, computer and privacy. What more could life throw at us? Over the years we built a relationship to count on. We listened, argued, criticized each other, laughed and cried within the safety net of a bond forged by blood and friendship.

As usual, we updated each other on our work lives and home lives. Stories saved from the week gone by were shared. I came close to telling him about my secret several times, but back then we did not have the relationship where a brother and sister could discuss the sister's IVF cycle. I kept the lid tightly closed on that jar.

As we were winding up, he said, 'By the way, I have something to tell you.'

'What?'

'I think Archana is pregnant.'

'Oh! Congratulations! When did you find out?'

'Today. She took a home pregnancy test and it is positive. We are planning to go to the doctor tomorrow.' He said the words casually, but there was excitement bubbling beneath the veneer of nonchalance. I asked all the routine questions.

'How is she feeling?'

'Does she have any symptoms?'

'Are you excited?'

Then, unable to control myself, I went technical, looking for any shred of evidence to poke holes in this pregnancy . . .

'How many days has it been since she missed her period?'

'Did she use the morning's first pee while taking the test?'

'Were the lines faint or dark?'

Gopal answered all these questions dutifully, without being suspicious of my advanced knowledge and interest in pregnancy testing. I put the phone down. The clock in my bedroom stopped ticking.

Gopal had married Archana two years ago. Ranjith and I had been married for six years. I was older to both Gopal and Archana. How could this be? To anyone who knew the rules of seniority, it should have been clear that *I* was supposed to get pregnant first. OK, fine, they were first off the mark, but what kind of timing was this? They had decided to get pregnant when my emotions, insecurities and hormones were in free fall. Was this the time of the year to have a baby? And

then, how was I going to give this news to the world? To my
in-laws? Could Gopal and Archana not think of my shame,
my pain in being the aberrant older sister? How in the world
could anyone be so insensitive? It was hard enough hearing
about my colleague Varsha's pregnancy, Sini's pregnancy,
Shahrukh Khan's surrogate baby. But now, in my own house
and family?

Ranjith reached earlier than expected, at four in the
afternoon. I had at last brushed my teeth, showered and made
the bed. He let himself into the house with his own key. As
he ambled into our bedroom, I was looking into a full-sized
mirror getting dressed to go out. This Sunday was intolerable.

I continued to comb my hair with my eyes still focused on
the mirror, barely acknowledging his presence.

'Archana is pregnant,' I said matter-of-factly.

He said nothing, sitting on the bed, looking at his phone.

'Don't you have anything to say?' I asked.

Still nothing.

I turned around, threw the comb on the bed and, hands
on hips, like a mother confronting a recalcitrant child, said,
'Don't you know what this means?'

'Yes. I do,' he said, looking up at me, 'You are shattered.'

14

To Double or Not to Double

Archana and Gopal visited a gynaecologist the next day. By evening the result of the beta hCG test was in—the value was 1500 mIU/ml! When I spoke to Gopal in the evening he was ignorant of what it meant. The normal range column in the report made it clear that Archana was pregnant; that was all that mattered to them. The gynaecologist waived the repeat test forty-eight hours later to check if the hCG was doubling. Gopal and Archana informed almost everyone in their respective families about the positive test, notwithstanding my advice for some reserve.

~

The two-week wait for my beta hCG had crossed the halfway mark—nine days over, five more to go. It was a Saturday evening and Ranjith and I walked to the Mall, situated on the main road about five hundred metres from our apartment. The Mall was our *adda,* and we strolled in wearing our flip-flops, hands in pockets, gazing at the shop windows decked up for Independence Day, which had just gone by. The building's facade was oddly shaped, half-circle, half-rectangle, and it jutted onto the main road like a poorly parked vehicle. It was not very big or upscale, attracting only the second- and third-tier retail brands, and the food court offered mostly standardized, ultra-processed fare that we avoided. But it was a familiar, intimate space for us. It was comforting to be lost in the midst of desultory shoppers, diners, movie-goers and hangers-on who seemed as aimless as us.

We did our regulation rounds of the three or four levels inside and returned home an hour later. I was sapped. Ranjith resumed his weekend job as a couch potato in front of the TV, flipping from Tamil comedy clips to Telugu comedy clips to Malayalam comedy clips. I retired to the bedroom, setting in motion the wheels of my IVF brain.

Tired? What did this mean?

The hormonal supplements I was on mimicked pregnancy symptoms, so it was not prudent to read too much into it. Besides, how much could I trust a symptom as vague as 'tiredness'? It was not specific to pregnancy, like sore breasts or night-time urination. But I had gone through IVF cycles before and had never experienced this level of fatigue. Maybe this cycle *had* worked. Maybe I *was* pregnant.

Should I take an HPT? Should I not? A long time was spent playing mental ping-pong with the idea. There was almost a week to go for the beta hCG, so if the HPT turned out to be negative it could be concluded that it was too early. Besides, why worry about a negative HPT? I had never seen a positive HPT in my life; this would be one more addition to that long line of dissenting tests.

Once a wicked thought strayed into my head it was impossible not to act on it.

HPTs mandate use of the morning's first urine because it is the most concentrated. Concentrated urine exhibits the highest levels of hCG, thereby rendering the test more accurate. I didn't want to wait until the next morning. I had not relieved myself since afternoon and decided to settle for four hours of hormonal consolidation.

Those days my bathroom always had a stash of HPTs. I tore open a new pack. There was no need to read the instructions leaflet. I dropped the urine sample and laid the white plastic case carefully on the washbasin counter. A single line appeared. I looked at myself in the mirror. *Nothing new.* Then, slowly, another line appeared. Fainter than the first, but there. I looked at myself in the mirror again, eyes widening, lips quivering. *Was this really happening?*

Storing the used HPT safely in the cupboard below the washbasin, I walked out as if nothing momentous had just occurred. I went back to bed but found it impossible to rest. I weighed my options. Should I tell Ranjith? Should I wait? How much should I rely on an HPT? We know what happened the last time I believed one. Should I risk making a fool of myself again?

An hour later, after dinner, Ranjith and I sat in the balcony adjoining our living room and overlooking a coconut tree plantation. I had convinced him that his commitment to the TV was touching but that every relationship needs some time away.

We chatted about this and that. A balmy breeze kept us company. My HPT secret was twisting and turning inside me. During a pause in the conversation, it made a getaway from my loosening grip. I confessed to Ranjith about the bathroom visit and the HPT.

He nodded his head.

He did not seem glad or surprised. Not even repeating or adding a 'Really?' to the piece of information I had just shared.

I looked fixedly at him for a few moments, expecting a delayed reaction. Nothing.

I was disappointed by this exhibition of supernatural calm, but the reasons were instinctively clear. A positive home pregnancy test was a good sign, but it was only the first step. It was like cutting the ribbon on the inauguration day of a store. It was just the beginning of an enterprise that had to last nine long months. This was not the time to lift me up, swirl me in the air and break into a song. Just because we had a positive HPT didn't mean we had a baby. It only meant that round one was ours.

There was no meaning in coaxing excitement out of him.

~

Every day after that I did an HPT to confirm that I was still pregnant. To my relief, the second pink line continued to surface. On Thursday, five days later, we went to the clinic for the first beta hCG test. The clinic called in the afternoon to reveal the result. The value was 142 mIU/mL. Now it was official. We did not feel any excitement, but were grateful for the quantitative proof of my pregnancy.

One of the reasons for our muted response to the news was the lab value itself. It was not an out-and-out win. I had tested positive on an HPT almost a week before. Even though the test didn't say it explicitly, I figured that the hCG value had to be at least 50 mIU/mL before it could be detected by an Indian HPT. So, if a week ago the hCG value was 50 mIU/mL, how could it be only 142 now? That meant it was *not* doubling every forty-eight hours as it should.

The team at the clinic was happy with the result, because seen as a standalone report it was no cause for concern. A starting beta hCG value of 142 mIU/mL was reason to celebrate, but Dr Leela did not know about my HPT adventures and I didn't dare tell her for fear of inviting rebuke. The test had to be repeated after two days to check if the beta hCG was doubling. If the next value was in excess of 280 mIU/ml, then we were on course.

I spent the next two days not fully convinced about the value, yet not entirely disappointed either, unsure about which box it went into. The box of triumphs or the box of debacles? I did not know then that this entire cycle would be an extended masterclass in liminality, spent in the twilight zone between success and failure.

~

On Saturday morning I gave the blood sample for the second beta hCG test and returned home. We expected to hear from the clinic by noon. There was a pattern in the way the clinic shared test results with patients. If you gave your blood sample at eight in the morning it took about three to four hours to run the test and share the result. If the news was bad the call came late. Maybe at one or sometimes as late as two. If the news was good the call came early, by twelve or sometimes even earlier. Anyway, I was not expecting bad news.

The clock struck twelve and the call was due any minute now. Maybe in the future a woman won't have to wait four hours to know the result of a beta hCG test. Perhaps a small prick of the skin would be enough to flash the value on a digital monitor, as with a glucometer. Maybe that blessing of technology is not too far away, but on that day there were no such substitutes. All we could do was ride out the suspense. The air in my house was still, cold and dense. Nothing moved. No one said a word. I lay curled up in bed, browsing the Internet aimlessly on my phone, unable to focus on any single page or piece of content. From head to toe my body was tingling with a shrill, nervous energy. Ranjith sat on the diwan in the living room working on his computer. I wondered more than once how he could type emails while standing on the edge of a precipice.

The minutes passed but the call did not come. By one, I supposed this was the undoing of another cycle. They would never delay a positive result so much, something was undoubtedly wrong. Sitting up on my bed, I called the hospital and found out that Dr Preetha was in a meeting and only she was authorized to share the result so we would have to wait. This made me feel marginally relieved. There was a non-medical explanation for why the result was delayed. Dr Preetha was probably stuck in some administrative hassle and hadn't been able to make the phone call. We continued to wait.

Another hour passed—still no call. They had never delayed even a negative result so much. I called the hospital again from my bed, sitting on my knees, elbows resting on a pillow in my lap. Dr Preetha was still not available.

'Can you just check if the result has been posted online? I just want to know if the beta hCG has doubled.' I pleaded with

Veena, the receptionist. I knew her well, having spent many hours in the waiting hall facing her. She had just come back to work post-maternity leave.

'Please,' I said again, trying to stoke compassion in her for a crumbling IVF patient.

'OK. But please don't tell Dr Preetha about it.'

'No, I won't.'

'Fine. What's your patient ID?'

'1514.'

I struggled to grip the phone with my moist hands as her fingers clicked keys on the computer.

She came back online in a few seconds and read out the number. The tense orchestra that was playing in our heads and had filled our entire house, ascending in volume and intensity, one note upon another, reached its climax and crashed to a stunning silence.

I thanked her and disconnected the call. Ranjith was standing next to me.

'It's 207,' I said. All the tension had evaporated in an instant, replaced by a sinking, weightless feeling.

'Hmm.'

'It hasn't doubled. It hasn't even come *close* to doubling.'

'I know.'

After a long pause, Ranjith shifted his attention to the practicalities of the afternoon.

'It's OK. Let's eat something. I will go out and get lunch.'

I continued to look away.

When I heard the door shut behind him, I buried my face in the pillow and burst into tears. Angry, sad, helpless tears.

Why couldn't just one thing go right? Just one number?

After some time I stopped. My eyes were red, cheeks wet and lungs aching. I wanted to talk to someone. Anyone. Just to share my anguish, to say it out loud. But it couldn't be Ranjith or my mother or anyone who really cared about me because I had to appear strong and unaffected before them. Who could it be then? Who was available on a Saturday afternoon to listen to my story of IVF heartbreak? Who was keen to learn about the abstruse world of doubling beta hCGs and vague HPTs? Even if someone was, did I have the patience to explain a textbook's worth of reproductive science before receiving a few ounces of succour? Besides, what could anyone say? At best, a facile, 'It's okay. It will happen. Don't worry.' No, it's *not* okay. And it *hasn't* happened. And the *worry* is all I have.

A beta hCG that climbs slowly or does not double in two or three days often indicates a failing pregnancy. My foetus was most likely on a mission to self-abort. But research on the Internet also showed that about 15 per cent of pregnancies may not adhere to this hCG doubling time frame and yet result in a perfectly healthy baby. I was back to square one. Did I belong to that 15 per cent cohort or did this just mean that miscarriage was imminent? Why couldn't the beta hCG *just* double? That would have been so much more convenient. If the value had not increased at all or had declined, the verdict would have been clear, one-sided, but now we were stuck between two floors in a claustrophobic elevator. Neither here nor there. Round two was inconclusive.

Dr Preetha called later that afternoon to communicate the result 'officially'. I pretended I was hearing it for the first time, by now having regained my composure. Dr Leela ordered a third beta hCG test four days later to clarify which direction this pregnancy was proceeding in and I applied for leave until then. There was no way I could focus on work with a sword hanging over my head.

~

Our fight against infertility began in a scientific, rational, problem-solving, data-driven mode. Which procedure? What protocol? Which drugs? What grades? These were the questions used to design and mount an attack against infertility. I was fond of saying to friends who suggested prayer or faith-based healing, 'If your car broke down in the middle of the road, what would you do? Call a mechanic or speak to God?' Infertility was essentially a mechanical problem which demanded a mechanical solution. Where was the scope for divine help?

At home, my mother and in-laws competed with each other to find new temples to offer prayers for a baby for us. We were advised to visit all the speciality temples from Rameshwaram to Mannarasala especially meant for childless couples. On these occasions I complied, but could not hide my contempt for the rituals. *Pushing an embryo through a catheter inside my uterus had failed. How was overturning a vessel going to help?*

When well-meaning elders implored me to pray more fervently for a child, assuming that there was some gap in my devotion, I defied their instructions. It seemed meaningless to drag God in to fix a very physical, practical, nuts-and-bolts kind of issue that had a ready answer in medicine. I was adamant about overcoming infertility without any divine intervention. A little nudge from science and it would work one of these days. But days passed, months passed, years passed. Yet we were no closer to having a baby than when I started treatment. Fertility medicine kept dangling the carrot of success in front of me and pulling away just when I thought I had grasped it.

As treatment progressed from IUIs to IVFs, from failed attempts to the last miscarriage, I began to rethink my sole reliance on medicine. The burden of success was on fertility medicine, but it became increasingly clear that medicine was entirely fallible. It could take the horse to water but could not make it drink. The best egg and the best sperm and the best endometrium were not guarantees for success. At the same time, a not-so-good egg and not-so-good sperm and not-so-good endometrium did not equate with failure. There was an unknown and unknowable element in childbirth. An element of luck. A small miracle in the making.

This was also not a fight to win through endurance, like losing weight or learning to swim. If you up the intensity of effort, at some stage you will drop the kilos or swim back-to-back laps, but I could submit myself to ten IVF cycles and still not have a baby. There was no point at which it *had* to work. This was a human endeavour with very little correlation between effort and outcome.

I was always indifferent to religion and to the idea of God. Amma and Achan did not demand adherence to any religious customs or even a daily prayer routine, despite Achan being a deeply devout man. We had a prayer room at home in Trivandrum that we were not allowed to enter with our slippers on. Every morning before going to the bank Achan sat down cross-legged on the floor in the puja room before half a dozen framed pictures of deities placed on a rosewood teapoy, lit an old silver lamp and incense sticks and spent half an hour reciting slokas and singing bhajans. But he never insisted that we participate. On Thursdays he offered more elaborate prayers in the evening. Even then we only joined him during *aarti* at the very end of the session. Gopal and I were disinterested, like most children and teenagers, eager to get back to whatever we were doing. There was neither a carefully studied rejection of religion nor an unquestioning embrace of it. We did not engage with it at all.

The first time I felt drawn towards religion and prayer was when I moved to Hyderabad to attend college. Feeling uprooted, I started visiting a nearby Malayalee Ayyappa temple every Saturday. It helped me stay connected with my past and my home in a city so far away from everything I knew. In the turmoil of hostel life, new friendships, new ways of reading and understanding, the temple offered constancy and stability. This practice continued as long as I stayed in Hyderabad. But once Ranjith and I got married and we moved to Bangalore, my temple visits became more erratic. There was no longer a need for maintaining a spiritual continuity with my past. It had merged with my present and I felt moored within the confines of a happy marriage.

Infertility was the second time in my life that I experienced the same psychic uprootedness. My rule book didn't apply any more—if you take the right medicine, you will be cured; if you work hard and persevere, you will most likely succeed; failure is always followed by success, etc. This was a province that operated outside this framework and I didn't know how to navigate it. Once a treatment cycle began, my mind was about as sturdy as a paper boat being tossed about in the high seas. One minute it was riding a wave, another minute it was drowning, and mostly it was coming apart. There was a dire need for something to hold on to, to find an inner balance, an unwavering core. And that need again led me to faith and God.

By the start of the current FET cycle, prayer had become an integral part of my everyday life. Every morning and evening I lit the lamp in the puja corner and repeated the same words seeking strength and guidance. Then I sat down with my laptop to listen to a series of slokas and devotional songs on YouTube, immersing myself in the reassurance provided by the lyrics. It became a therapeutic tool to deal with the psychological pressures of IVF. Daily prayer calmed my nerves and gave me the confidence that a higher power was watching over me, something that transcended the natural laws. This act of surrender allowed me to transfer the burden of success to something other-worldly, to ease my own sense of responsibility towards the outcome. I certainly did not expect to have a child because I was *now* expressing my devotion to God. But that devotion provided me the emotional scaffolding to keep sailing in a treacherous sea.

The IVF process consisted of several blocks of time, such as the two-week wait, the wait for the beta hCG test result or the wait for the ultrasound, when all action was suspended and there was no visibility of progress inside the body. During such phases, prayer became an effective means to expand my trust and believe that everything was going as planned. The three days that I had to last between the second and third beta hCG tests was one such example. I repeatedly invoked 'Krishna Guruvayurappa', urging the god to come to my rescue. This prayer helped me pull through those seventy-two hours as well as stay somewhat steady through the rise and fall of fortunes that infertility and its treatment entailed.

~

On Wednesday we went to the clinic for the third beta hCG test, four days after the last test. It was Janmashtami. I had more or less come to terms with the idea that this pregnancy too was over and was preparing myself mentally to go to office from the next day. Working from home had extended to almost three and a half weeks now and I wanted to get this ritual over with before moving on with the rest of my life, which had been suspended for the sake of a slithery pregnancy.

I sat on the chair arranged perpendicular to the table in the nurses' station and extended my arm.

Sini was her usual sunny self. While drawing the blood into the syringe, she said, 'Let's hope that the value is more than 600.'

I was shocked. Did she still harbour hopes from this cycle?

But instead of saying that, my mouth instinctively uttered, 'Naakku ponn aavatte.' Let's hope what you are saying turns out to be true.

Ranjith left for office directly from the hospital and I went home, switched off my phone and forced myself to go to sleep. It was nine in the morning but I did not want to contend with any of the units of time that made up the next three hours.

At eleven, I stirred from bed and began pottering about the house. After about half an hour I started wondering about the test results. No one had called. Then I realized that my phone was still switched off. When I switched on my phone there were missed calls from Ranjith and the hospital. I called the clinic, but the line was engaged. I called Ranjith. He sounded worried.

'I have been trying to reach you. What were you doing?'

'Nothing. I was sleeping. The phone was off.'

'OK. Since the clinic couldn't get through to you, they called me. The results are in.'

'Hmm.'

'Guess what?'

'What?'

'The value is 680!'

'Whaaat?'

The beta hCG, which hadn't doubled in the first forty-eight hours, had now shot up by almost five times from the original value. Instead of doubling neatly every two days, it had chosen to take it easy at first and then shoot up the charts. My hormones craved drama.

I got dressed in a jubilant, tearful hurry and drove myself to the clinic to get supplementary hormonal shots. I thanked Sini again and again for mouthing those words that turned out to be prophetic. It was one of those rare days when I felt the presence of a benevolent force in my life. Was this the miracle that I was waiting for? Was this a sign that everything would be bright and clear from here on? Whatever it was, I felt blessed. We were still not out of the woods. The ultrasound scheduled two weeks later would give us a clearer picture about the pregnancy, but at least round three was ours, hook, line and sinker.

15

How Many Beats Per Minute?

Gopal and Archana went for the first ultrasound to assess foetal viability at eight weeks. The next day Gopal posted a video in the family email group. The subject line said, 'Our baby's heartbeat.' I did a double take when I saw that phrase, startled by the certainty and confidence in his words. He was sure that there was a baby arriving at the end of this pregnancy, he was sure enough to define the foetus as 'our baby', to boast and declare that ownership. Hadn't he heard of ends that came before their time? I avoided opening that email for a while. Eventually my curiosity got the better of me and I opened it. He had made a recording on his phone of the black-and-white monitor which displayed the foetal heart rate. It was 179 beats per minute. A strong, healthy heart.

Gopal and Archana knew about my pregnancy from Amma, but we never brought it up with each other. It was an open secret. If the pregnancy continued and normalized, it would be openly acknowledged. If it failed to progress, the 'secrecy' spared both parties the awkwardness of explanations.

~

Our lives continued to play out in two-week modules, as we held our breath from one milestone to another. I resumed working from home, leaving my manager to wonder if she should assign my workstation to another team member. Colleagues had been told that I was going through some 'health issues' to explain my continued absence. Word about my pregnancy must have spread in the gossip circles, but I was sheltered from all contact with humanity, the only exceptions being visits to temples on weekends. There was a daily routine of prayer, work and rest that I adhered to with monk-like discipline. As long as I stayed at home and repeated this cycle without any disruptions, I believed I was safe. Not too long ago, this pregnancy had looked like a speeding car destined to meet a waiting disaster. But against all odds, the brakes slammed, the wheels screeched, and the car made a U-turn at the very last minute. I owed it to whatever force that was directing this sequence of events to stay positive and happy. We had come this far. We would get through the rest too.

We reached the first ultrasound mark without any further hiccups. Patients continue to visit the IVF clinic for ultrasounds and other investigations even after pregnancy is confirmed. The risk of miscarriage is highest in the first twelve weeks, and therefore IVF pregnancies are subject to more intense monitoring during this period. For an IVF pregnancy, ultrasounds are scheduled at six weeks, eight weeks and then twelve weeks. Once the twelve-week barrier is crossed, the patient is ready to be 'mainstreamed'. At three months, you get to graduate and move to the main hospital and join other 'naturally' pregnant women. You are assigned the pink-and-white hospital folder of antenatal care with the photograph of a tranquil woman cradling her belly on the front cover. It said, 'Happy Motherhood'. Until then I had to be content with my overflowing blue file of the fertility centre, which I carried around hidden inside a plastic shopping bag.

At the clinic, when it was my turn, I went to the bathroom, removed my salwar and panties, hung them on the steel rod and lay on the bed. The radiologist came in. At seven weeks and five days we expected to see the gestational sac and foetal pole and detect some cardiac activity. Of these, the foetal heartbeat was the most critical. If a heartbeat is detected, the odds of the pregnancy progressing significantly improve. I was praying with every fibre and nerve in my body for a foetal heartbeat. Once I heard the heartbeat, I thought I was through.

Dr Sushma was an experienced radiologist and served the fertility clinic exclusively. Since I started coming to the clinic, she had gone through pregnancy, childbirth, maternity leave and had even rejoined hospital duties, while I had not budged an inch from my position in the fertility line. She asked for the date of my last menstrual period and began to do her job in a competent yet aloof manner. I chanted 'Krishna Guruvayurappa' non-stop in my head. After a couple of minutes, she made her first remark, 'I think this pregnancy has implanted late.' The chanting was cut short.

She could visualize the sac, foetus and heartbeat, but none of the three corresponded with the stage of pregnancy I was in. The length of the foetus was only 3.6 mm, which corresponded to six weeks (I was seven weeks, five days pregnant). The gestational age of the foetus was more than ten days behind schedule. The heart rate was only 108 beats per minute (bpm). Anything above 120 bpm was considered normal at this stage. There was a live foetus inside my uterus but neither its growth nor its heart rate matched the date of the pregnancy.

I got dressed, went back to the waiting hall and relayed to Ranjith what Dr Sushma had told me. It was exasperating. If there had been no foetus or a cripplingly low heart rate, we could have formed a definitive conclusion. But now all we could do was wait and watch to see if foetal growth and heart rate picked up pace or halted midway. We were again grounded in an indeterminate zone, neither in nor out.

There was a long queue of patients waiting to meet Dr Leela and we were anxious to hear her opinion. When our turn came at last, Dr Leela took us by surprise. She did not seem concerned about the growth lag or the slow heart rate. I didn't know if she was just posturing so that I wouldn't worry or if she genuinely didn't think it was a problem.

'The heart rate will climb up. Let's do another ultrasound a week later to check,' she said unconcernedly.

When I went back to the nurse's station and cross-checked with Sini, she was even more dismissive of my concerns.

'Once the heartbeat has been detected, you have nothing to worry. It always starts out low and then increases week on week,' she assured me.

I could not completely squash the niggling doubts in my head, but I was determined to stay positive, drawing faith from their words. Ranjith and I decided to stop at Adiga's for filter coffee and idli-vada, having skipped breakfast at home.

Sitting in the mostly empty, heavily upholstered service area, I tried hard to be grateful and happy for the onward movement, but the low heart rate loomed large. Should I take Dr Leela's and Sini's words at face value? Would the heart rate really climb up as they claimed? Or was this another miscarriage-in-waiting? At each stage, I sought certitude, a clear prediction about the future, and it kept evading me. The more I craved for firmness of outcome, the more indefinite the progress seemed. It was the life of a contestant on a reality show who must stave off the threat of elimination week after week. It was the *very* format of the show to keep me on edge—there was no point in looking for serenity.

~

In the intervening week between the first and the second ultrasound, my mother and grandmother were expected to visit us on their annual Bangalore trip. Their tickets were booked three months ago, much before this pregnancy was anywhere on the horizon. Given the dicey state of affairs, I did not feel particularly thrilled at the prospect of having them over. This pregnancy was turning out to be a slow, strenuous climb uphill, and I was not in the shape to host house guests, cook feasts for them and take them out on day tours (I know, they were my own mother and grandmother). But for Amma and Ammamma a visit to Bangalore was a 'vacation', and they expected resort-style treatment with welcome drink, buffet and sightseeing. They were coming here to spend time with us, but they were also coming here to 'party'.

Ammamma retired as principal of one of the oldest and largest (in terms of student size) government schools in the state after a long career in teaching. She was a measured, thoughtful person who put off the smallest of decisions because she wanted more time to deliberate. She spent her time reading history and fiction in Malayalam and English. Before she took her afternoon nap she listened to news on the radio. And her evenings were spent glued to the mega-serials on Malayalam channels, which she admitted were obnoxious. Her days had the steady, meandering pace of a river at peace with itself. In comparison, Amma was a breakaway boulder rolling downhill in a mad, blind hurry. She wanted to be everywhere and do everything. Her days were packed with relentless activity and fraternizing, squeezing in as many weddings, funerals, house-warming ceremonies, residents' association meetings and alumni get-togethers into a span of twenty-four hours as was humanly possible. She visited exhibitions and flea markets, buying knickknacks no one had any use for. She made excuses to host friends and colleagues for breakfast and high tea, using these occasions to flaunt all the recipes she had learnt from food shows on TV.

Their diametrically opposite personalities caused daily friction. The most innocuous of remarks had the potential to blow up into an all-out war, and we were more than a little wary about their cohabitation. But despite all their differences there was one thing that brought them together—a common love for people, company and conversation. Amma and Ammamma found it unnatural to sit through a flight or train journey without interrogating their fellow passengers. In Trivandrum, the front door of our house was opened at six in the morning, and the wooden doorstop wedged in the hinge. It was unseated from this position only in the afternoon when Ammamma took her nap. By four in the afternoon the doorstop was back in place and Ammamma sat in the veranda to welcome neighbours, friends, acquaintances and anyone else who passed by. Snacks were served, gossip shared, and political views clarified. To be shut inside a two-bedroom flat all day was equivalent to hypoxia. Therefore, before coming to Bangalore, Amma and Ammamma dutifully rang up all their contacts in the city and made plans to visit or be visited.

The furthest extent of my socializing lay in recognizing and greeting those who lived next door when encountered in the lift. Weddings, excursions and New Year's Eve parties were the substance of nightmares. When Ranjith labelled me the 'original anti-social', I blushed with pride. I thrived on solitude; Amma and Ammamma thrived on society. In the normal course of events I would have made the necessary personality and lifestyle adjustments for the week or ten days that they stayed with us and resigned myself to a people overdose. But, in the middle of my second pregnancy, my bandwidth was already worn thin. I saw myself as a crusader on a mission that tottered dangerously between life and death. This was not the time for social niceties.

There were other reasons too. My mother knew I was pregnant, Ammamma didn't. I was not yet ready to tell her or anyone else because of my fluctuating pregnancy graph. If the zigzag line steadied by the next ultrasound, it could be disclosed. In the meantime, I did not want to disturb the isolation of my cocoon. I was also superstitious. The last time someone visited us during my pregnancy, I miscarried. Should I invite misfortune again? I felt I had good reasons to beg off this visit. In fact, I had every intention of saying to Amma, 'Please can you visit another time. I don't think I

can or want to deal with this right now.' Instead, I ended up
saying, 'Sure. Come over. It's fine.'

~

Despite Dr Leela's assurances and my stated intent to be calm
and relaxed, at heart I could not stop worrying. Dr Sushma's
late-implantation theory did not hold water. There was a
very narrow margin for ambiguity as far as implantation was
concerned. We knew exactly which day the eight-cell embryos
were placed in the uterus, and they had to implant in the next
three to four days. Further, I had tested positive on an HPT
just a week after the transfer. So this couldn't be a case of late
implantation at all. And if it was so, then what did one make
of the low foetal heart rate (FHR)? A private investigation
began on Google.

At seven weeks the normal FHR is equal to or greater than
120 bpm. My foetal heart rate at the ultrasound was only 108
bpm. I came upon a study[1] on Google Scholar that evaluated
pregnancies at six to eight weeks to determine the relationship
between heart rate and first trimester outcome. In the group the
study examined, *all* embryos with heart rates below 110 bpm at
seven to eight weeks died. Please note, *all*. My foetal heart rate
was 108 bpm at seven weeks. We were short by two heartbeats,
by the margin of two delicate flutters of a still-forming heart.

When the gist of the paper hit me, my stomach dropped.
If what the paper was saying was true, we were on the path

---

[1] P.M. Doubilet and C.B. Benson, 'Embryonic Heart Rate in the Early First
Trimester: What Rate Is Normal?', *Journal of Ultrasound in Medicine* vol.
14, no.6 (June 1995): 431–34, https://doi.org/10.7863/jum.1995.14.6.431.

to inevitable foetal demise. I wondered how much weightage and credence I should give to the conclusions of the research study. Were there any loopholes in their methodology? Was the finding an immutable truth or was there some margin for error? I didn't know. I wondered if I was going to break all the rules of reproductive medicine and make it past the first trimester or if I would just end up further underlining the rule. Nothing was in my command. I resolved to rest as much as I could to increase the flow of blood to the uterus, hoping that would keep the baby's heart beating. I also prayed. The rest was up in the air, out of the reach of any human hand.

~

Amma and Ammamma's trip fell in the middle of Onam, our most anticipated festival. In Kerala, for the ten days that Onam celebrations lasted, the entire state transformed itself into a giant carnival, with community banquet lunches, flower rangolis, illuminated streets and buildings, floats and tableaux, cultural performances, food melas, handicraft exhibitions and more. In not-so-distant Bangalore, there was no scent of the gaiety that swept up Kerala. In a feeble attempt to rev up atmosphere on Thiruvonam day, I switched on the TV and turned up the volume first thing in the morning. The Onam advertisements, Onam special movies and the Onam greetings on Malayalam TV channels delivered some of the festival frolic home. Without TV, there was hardly any Onam in Bangalore.

We made the *sadhya* and drew up an amateur *pookalam* on the living room floor. Ammamma's sister who lived in Bangalore joined us in the afternoon for the traditional feast.

After lunch Ammamma went back with her to spend a few days in her house. A collective sigh rose once we saw them off. We could now drop the act and openly address the elephant in the room—my pregnancy.

For the next two days Amma took the reins of the kitchen and I stopped any show of help, lazing around until my meals were hand-delivered to the couch in front of the TV. It was comforting to have someone else in the house, someone who was not clued into the intricacies of this pregnancy the same way Ranjith and I were. It was comforting to share her slightly distant, fuzzy gaze. Unlike us, Amma was calm and relaxed and talked about the regular goings-on in the family and the world. There was no guillotine suspended above her neck.

The week passed uneventfully. There had been no signs of a miscarriage, and the so-called pregnancy symptoms were all in place (bouts of giddiness, enhanced veins on my breast and a ravenous appetite). It looked as if we were all set to hit the second ultrasound mark without any unwanted excitement. However, the night before the ultrasound was due, a sharp stabbing sensation in my abdomen woke me up from sleep. I howled in pain, waking up Ranjith before lurching towards the bathroom. I was positive that there would be blood in my panties and this would be the catastrophic end to another pregnancy. But in the white light of the bathroom, the panties were clean. There was no blood. *What was that pain then? It was strong enough to jolt me out of sleep.*

I rolled back in bed, spooning against Ranjith, scared to animate even a finger. He kept saying, 'It's fine. Nothing will happen,' holding my hands tightly, trying to hush the thud of my rapidly beating heart. My eyes were open for some time expecting more pain. But there was none, and I fell asleep.

In the morning when I arose, I lost no time in going to the bathroom to check for blood. Again, in clear daylight, there was none. I relaxed. We had made it this far. We would get through the rest too.

Amma made my favourite grilled sandwiches for breakfast. I wore my lucky green kurta and lucky green earrings and faithfully completed the morning ritual of prayers, dabbing a line of bhasmam on my forehead for extra luck. Amma came to the lift to see us off before we headed to the clinic.

~

I have taken multiple stabs at writing what happened next, trying to build suspense and anxiety about the outcome of the ultrasound, extracting as much as I can from this emotional coal mine—the probe inside my vagina, the look on the doctor's face, my trembling self, and such. But I think I am done with the drama, with building pathos. Done with the exhausting twists and turns of my infertility saga. Let's go all matter-of-fact and technical. Besides, don't we already know how that day turned out? Aren't there enough layperson lessons on reproductive medicine to suggest that? What are the odds of a pregnancy with a beta hCG that fails to double? What are the chances of a pregnancy with a foetal heart rate lower than 110 bpm at seven weeks? What is the likelihood of such a pregnancy progressing? The correct answer is, NIL. I was a fugitive trying to run away with my illusions, but eventually reality caught up and dragged me back to its ramparts, bound, gagged, kicking and screaming. This pregnancy had nowhere to go but down.

It was a silent miscarriage. The foetus had died but the body had failed to identify the loss, resulting in an asymptomatic abortion. The baby's heart had stopped beating sometime in the middle of the night before the ultrasound—that was the exact point Dr Sushma nailed down for foetal demise. She said it had to be very recent because the foetus had almost doubled in size since the last scan. The pain that I felt the previous night was perhaps my baby's last cry, a cry that escaped her throat even though she meant to leave quietly, without warning, without farewell.

I gave Amma the news on the phone from the clinic but did not want to inform my grandmother, who remained ignorant about the pregnancy and its loss. Amma was warned against bringing this up ever again. I was never pregnant and never miscarried. But there was one open question we had to resolve before the embargo. Amma had unearthed a long-lost relative in Bangalore and had set up dinner with his family for the next day. I had last seen him when I was five years old and when he was still a bachelor. Now he had a daughter near my age.

'Should we go ahead with it or call it off? What do you think?' she asked, genuinely seeking direction.

I had every intention of saying, 'Yes, please call it off. Do you even need to ask?', but when the words came out, they sounded like, 'Yes. It's fine. Let's go ahead.' *A dinner party with a dead baby in your stomach. What's there to ask?*

Ranjith felt he owed it to his parents to share news of the miscarriage even though they did not know about the pregnancy. They were obviously miffed about the lapse in communication. My mother-in-law claimed that she suspected I was pregnant because she had spotted a kite in the temple compound adjacent to her house a week ago. Spotting a kite apparently means someone in your family is pregnant.

They asked us why we hadn't been more careful. Ranjith tried to explain that our caution or lack of caution had nothing to do with it. But I think the miscarriage registered with them mostly as a consequence of our negligence and carelessness. *How can you lose pregnancies again and again?*

After a repeat ultrasound two days later, to reconfirm foetal death, I went to the nurse's station to bid farewell to Sini. I didn't think our paths would cross again. She was going on maternity leave the next month and it was not certain if she would come back to work after the baby. All I managed to say was 'All the best', hoping it communicated all the gratitude and affection that I felt for her.

Five days after the miscarriage, after Amma and Ammamma had left for Trivandrum, I got admitted for a D&C (dilation and curettage). Since this pregnancy had progressed to almost nine weeks, Dr Leela suggested it was better to opt for a surgical removal of pregnancy tissue rather than induce an abortion, which might cause heavy bleeding and pain. I signed up for D&C thinking it would be quick and easy. The procedure was posted for eight in the morning in the operating theatre's schedule. Ranjith and I checked ourselves into a hospital room the previous night. At around two in the morning, the duty doctor and nurse came into the room, switched on the lights and woke me up.

'I am going to insert a suppository inside for the D&C,' the doctor explained.

When she was done depositing the tablet inside my vagina, she warned, 'There might be little pain, a little pain like your periods.'

A buzzer went off in my brain. There was nothing 'little' about period pain, for which I used Meftal-Spas every month.

I was right. As the suppository began to melt and infiltrate my blood stream, the contractions kicked in. At first I rolled from side to side on the bed, arms locked against my belly to manage the pain. Then I made visits to the bathroom to empty my bowels and throw up the previous night's dinner. Then I begged for pain relief. The staff refused. It was only a 'little pain', remember? So the 'little pain' continued for the next six hours until I was put under in the operating theatre, squeezed dry and bloodless, ready to cave into the blank sleep of anaesthesia. I told myself, 'We have come this far. We will get through the rest too.'

~

The same evening, I was discharged. Ranjith and I drove back home. An invisible yet palpable fog of pain hung above us. We stopped to pick up dinner from a fast-food restaurant on the way. When we reached our building Ranjith stopped the car near the basement elevator so that I could get off, before going ahead to park. I dragged my body and my mind, which felt sore on so many levels, to our sixth-floor apartment, turned on the lights and went to the bedroom to change. It took Ranjith eleven minutes to come. I didn't call to check, because I knew. A man deserves at least eleven minutes of privacy inside a parked car to drain his heartache.

I heard a knock on the bedroom door. When I opened it he walked past me without looking and sat down on the edge of the bed, facing the balcony. He buried his face in his hands and sobbed again. A deep, guttural sob.

I sat down on the bed and watched the tears of a broken man. The tears of someone whose last dregs of innocence, faith and hope have been emptied. I watched helplessly the impossible cruelty of that sight. He cried without being able to stop, without knowing why the crying won't stop. Really, I don't think he ever stopped crying.

16

Mother Knows Best

Before I met Ranjith I had been on the arranged marriage circuit for many months. I was rejected by some and I rejected some. When I was rejected I heaved a quiet sigh of relief and suppressed a half-smile while trying to appear heartbroken. Being rejected meant that I didn't have to do any explaining at home. The man had exercised his sole and exclusive privilege and saved me the hassle of convincing my parents why I chose to reject someone. My mother believed that if any man condescended to accept me as his wife then I should immediately fall to the ground, kiss his feet and thank the almighty for this windfall of fortune. I should then run to the nearest marriage hall or temple, whichever came first, and proceed to get married at the next available *muhurtam*. The idea that *I* may not like someone and therefore not wish to marry him was too ridiculous to consider. So if I had to reject a man ('boy'), it was like arguing at the Supreme Court for the death penalty. The circumstances had better be exceptionally revolting, exceedingly brutal and diabolical; only the 'rarest of rare' cases warranted such an extreme step. Frivolous arguments such as 'we don't have any common interests' or 'he wants us to live with his parents' or 'he wants me to quit my job and move to Kochi' were not acceptable.

In the initial days I made rookie mistakes, saying outright, 'No, I don't like this man. I don't want to marry him.' My frank and honest approach impressed no one, Amma least of all. My statement would set in motion an emotional juggernaut comprising hours of argument, blackmail, tears, then silence, then some more tears and silence. She would point out my considerable limitations and the Himalayan task of finding a suitor for a 'girl' who was too tall (75 per cent of the catchment was automatically disqualified because of this), too old (at twenty-five, most software engineers have planned their grandchildren) and not professionally qualified. I had studied neither engineering nor medicine. Of what use could I be in my marital home?

Over time, my strategies were sharpened and an arsenal of weapons prepared for a counterstrike. I would say, 'I need some time to think. I want to meet him a few more times and get to know him better before making up my mind.' This sounded reasonable and my mother agreed, her hopes rising. I was counting on the prospective groom saying or doing something in the second or third meeting which would help my case. Sometimes, after the fifth meeting, when I was still buying time, the boy's family would get annoyed at my delaying tactics and back off themselves. Or I would make a request: 'I want to go to the US to do a PhD. Can we get married after five years? Is that too long?' The singular objective was to get the man to say 'No'. I don't know if the credit goes to my tenacity and manoeuvring or to the fact that at heart Amma empathized with what I was saying. But in her urgency to get me married she was willing to overlook my consent. Eventually, good sense prevailed, the train wreck was averted and peace returned—for about twelve to fifteen minutes, until the next profile of a 'Simple, humble, Nair boy with no bad habits' from Bharat Matrimony hit our sphere.

I met Ranjith because I had nothing to do on a Sunday. I was all alone in my apartment in Hyderabad and thought meeting a potential suitor would be more compelling than doing the dishes or folding my clothes (by now I had moved out of the paying guest facility). Not having the energy to ward off another proposal from my mother, I thought it would be faster to just swallow the pill. I had budgeted for an hour, an hour and a half at the most, and picked Minerva Coffee Shop—a short distance from where I stayed—for our meeting.

Minerva Coffee Shop was an upmarket version of a Darshini—vegetarian south Indian food, quick service and reasonable pricing. I wanted to keep this as short and quick as possible, with minimum damage to the purse and psyche. I intended to go to a temple afterwards, come back and eat leftovers from the previous day's takeaway for dinner. My evening plans were cleverly laid out.

By four I began to feel restless at home and decided to get dressed. I chose a black-and-maroon cotton kurta with a Chinese collar that accentuated my slim waist, made my broad shoulders look narrow and covered my flabby arms. I put on eyeliner and lip gloss and tied my hair in a ponytail, arriving at that delicate balance between not too casual and not too dressed up. I flagged down a rickshaw and left for the coffee shop half an hour in advance because I didn't want to dirty the utensils at home making my evening tea.

The previous evening on the phone, when we spoke to each other to decide the venue, he seemed as disinterested as I was, leaving the time of day and choice of restaurant to my preferences. He was playing a cricket match and was padded up to bat next. He didn't want to use up any more minutes than was strictly necessary. I felt confident that this was going to be a quick and clean affair with little to no emotional fallout. If everything went well, he would tell his parents *first* that I was not his dream girl.

At Minerva, I chose the sofa-end of a corner table in the airconditioned section, ordered filter coffee and checked the front door from the periphery of my vision. At five he walked in. As soon as I spotted the face from the photograph emailed earlier, my eyes widened and pulse quickened, and there was the distinct pop of my 'plans' blowing up in a shower of confetti. All bets were off.

We shook hands, introduced ourselves and sat down. He ordered mini-idlis, I another round of coffee. There was no way I was going to eat in front of a man I wanted to impress. We began talking about our jobs, commutes, interests and the like. Within ten minutes of the conversation, I was leaning forward halfway across the table, unable to contain my burgeoning enthusiasm for this person I had just met. I stopped myself and leaned back, dialling down my fervour a notch or two. Why display such open interest in the very first meeting?

Well, what was his heart-stopping appeal?

He wore a blue linen shirt with a pair of denims (one point for good taste!).

He watched Lonely Planet and Ian Wright was his favourite travel show presenter. We both loved the episode on Mongolia.

(*Please note, this was 2006, before a hundred thousand shows on food and travel had descended on Indian television.*)

He said, 'I am absolutely materialistic', in the very first meeting with heart-winning candour.

When I suggested I wanted to go abroad for higher studies, he said, 'Fine, I will come with you.' (I still harboured hopes of studying in a foreign university.)

He made Malayalam sound sexy though he uttered only two words of it, one of which was technically English. 'Late *aayo?*'

He was tall and lean, curly-haired and freckle-faced, a solitary dimple peeking every now and then from his right cheek.

But most of all, he was the owner of the world's best smile. This is a smile worth having all to myself, I thought.

At his end, the only standout observation about me was that I was sufficiently different from him to pique his interest. He thought it would be madly exciting to be with someone who seemed his antithesis. He was an engineer; I came from the arts. His favourite author was Louis L'Amour; I swooned over Neruda's poetry. He had grown up in Kolar about a hundred kilometres from Bangalore and knew very little about his home state. I was born and raised in Kerala and knew very little about the world outside. Of course, he lived to regret the above-mentioned points about me, which soon turned from novelties to irritants. But now we are getting ahead of ourselves.

For the first time in my life, I grasped what it is to fall in love, to get to know a man in parts and then fall in love with each new part. Each day was an impatient biding of time until we could meet. We walked aimlessly along the Hussain Sagar, seeing afresh the planned gardens, shiny roads and city lights around us. We drove in his car all night, swapping stories and stopping for midnight tea served in pint-sized plastic cups by tea-sellers on bicycles. Some nights, we stayed back in my apartment, cooking dinner, talking, losing ourselves in the first explorations of desire, negotiating back and forth over when he would leave. On weekends we stayed over at his flat, settling down on a mattress dragged to the living room floor even though the house had two bedrooms and two cots in each. We woke up late on Sundays, ordered brunch and took turns reading *Calvin and Hobbes* and Pablo Neruda's poetry to each other.

He walked in and wiped my slate clean, brought down walls that had taken years to build and entered my being, seeping into every crevice and cavity until we were one and the same, unable to tell each other apart.

To keep things short, I did not go to the temple that day or eat the previous day's leftovers for dinner. I did not go abroad for higher studies. In fact, I ran to the nearest marriage hall and got married at the next available muhurtam. Well, what do they say? A mother always knows best.

17

Are You on Treatment?

Weeks drifted by. Life picked itself up and started walking again. The hospital folder was stashed back in the pull-out drawers underneath our bed. Strips of half-consumed pills were scissored and dropped in the trash can. The bleeding stopped, even the crying stopped. Hands and feet found their rhythm. The mind regained its edge. But the heaviness refused to lift. It was in my gait, my skin, my eyes. Dragging me down like the force of gravity itself, never letting me forget the weight of my defeat—an all-pervasive reminder of the futility of hope, prayers and dreams.

~

A month after the second miscarriage we travelled to Ottappalam to attend Ranjith's cousin's wedding. We reached the town the day before the wedding on a Saturday. Ranjith was running a fever and spent all day resting in one of the rooms, while guests milled around in all other parts of the house. I was worried about him, but I couldn't be seen clinging to my husband in front of his family. I did the best I could, not being very adept at the art of making myself useful on such occasions. I served juice in paper cups to newly arriving batches of guests, helped in serving the umpteen dishes on the *sadhya* leaf and reached out to aged aunts and uncles even though I was not quite sure how they were related to us. On the wedding day I draped myself in the silk saree that I had worn for my own wedding reception, decked myself in adequate gold jewellery and followed the bride to the pandal along with the other girls holding the *thaalam*. In my mind I was scoring well on the daughter-in-law index.

After the wedding, Ranjith and I were among the others who accompanied the bride to her new husband's home. In this house overflowing with guests too, we parked ourselves wherever space was available. At some point I was alone in a bedroom with one of Ranjith's relatives. I did not know her too well, but I held her in high regard. Her husband had lost his mobility a few years ago because of an autoimmune disorder. She ran the house single-handedly, took care of her husband confined to his bed and raised her children in a manner that gave no one an inkling of the burden she carried. She maintained cordial ties with her husband's family, making it a point to join every ceremony. I felt some solidarity with her. She too, like me, was an outsider in the family, a daughter-in-law.

So, in that post-wedding buzz, we were alone in a room deserted momentarily by the floating crowd. We sat on the edge of the bed strewn with wedding gifts, an awkward silence brewing between us. I was racking my brain for small talk when, without any forewarning, she asked me softly, 'Are you on treatment?' I should have laughed out aloud at the irony.

After four IUIs, two IVF cycles, an FET and two miscarriages! *Are you on treatment?* Instead, I went blank, the familiar dread of being caught, exposed, rising up my stomach.

I made some noise and looked away, displaying my discomfiture.

She kept her eyes on me for some time, expecting more information. Eventually, she too looked away. The awkward silence was now an impregnable wall.

A voice announced that it was time for tea and we both got up and went our separate ways. I sought out Ranjith and she went missing in the crowd. But her words were echoing in my head like a jammed tape. *Are you on treatment?*

We did not know each other well enough for such an intimate and probing question. We had only met a handful of times on occasions such as this. I didn't remember ever sitting down one-on-one to have a conversation with her. Yet, she had asked the question she did. It seemed as if she had been waiting for this quiet moment and as soon as an opportunity presented itself, she popped the question. She did not initiate pleasantries or build any context. She did not ask about my life, work or routine. This was the only thing about me that stood out for her. This was the only question she found worthy of asking me. *Why are you not pregnant and what are you doing about it?*

Since we had been married for over six years by then, she assumed there was something wrong enough warranting treatment. Hearing the word 'treatment' from somebody else made me feel like I had a disease (I know this book is inundated with that word). Infertility was not an affliction. It was not cancer or typhoid or arthritis with painful symptoms which had to be 'cured' by medicine to return the body to its normal state of being. Infertility had no palpable presence inside my body, it could only be defined by absence, the absence of conception. In fact, academics have posited that infertility, unlike many other medical conditions, is a social construct. It presupposes the aspiration for children. Without this aspiration there is no infertility. When the condition itself had such a wobbly premise, why was I being made to feel like a sick person? And moreover, I was not 'infertile' on my own. A specific combination of man and woman had not succeeded so far in producing a child. But that could change tomorrow and quite possibly without any medical intervention either.

I didn't know what she expected me to say in response. Did she want me to say, 'Yes, we are undergoing treatment', so that she could be satisfied that we were addressing the condition and that it would be alleviated soon? Or did she expect me to confess instantly about the procedures and share details of our failures and successes? Or did she expect me to say 'No, not yet, can you point us to a good doctor?' I have no idea what would have been the right thing to say. This was not the first time I had encountered such a seemingly innocuous query. This was not the last time either, but I never learnt to ignore it, to swat it like a pesky fly. It got me every time. Every time I felt reduced. My faculties, experiences, actions, reduced to a single all-hinging, all-determining question mark. Are you pregnant? If not, why not?

It dawned on me that I could achieve any level of professional success, social standing or personal growth, but the defining yardstick that would be used to measure my worth would be whether I had children or not. If I continued to remain childless, I would be described by that caveat, '*But she has no children*', inviting the 'oohs' and 'aahs' of sympathy and patronizing compassion. Perhaps inviting an additional comment, '*Enthu indayittu entha? Kuttikallu illa.*' What's the use of anything she has? No children. Having no children nullified and overruled everything else, making the one with child feel instantaneously superior.

I was not keen to be the recipient of this pity, the carrier of this incapacity; the odd one, the unlucky one. I wanted to climb over this fence and cross over to the other side where I would be like everyone else, a mother. My assets and liabilities level with those of everyone else.

Surely, I had enough education and exposure to dismiss these opinions. To know that not having a child did not subtract anything from me. While it was desirable to have a child for the joys and pains that parenting brought, just becoming a parent held no warranty of making me a better, more complete or worthy person. But it's one thing to know something in your head and another to live it. All the feminist theory from my postgraduate course could not come to my rescue when I needed it. I displayed neither the boldness to interject one of these conversations and point out that having a child could not be the touchstone of someone's value nor the insouciance to just leave things as they are without explaining anything or seeking approval. And this need to belong, the need to scrunch and squeeze myself into the mould as fully as possible, became one of my strongest motivations to overcome infertility.

Because this need for acceptance and affiliation was so fierce, when motherhood was denied to me it tore through my self-esteem and confidence. I questioned my own worthiness to have a child. Maybe my intentions were not 'pure' and sincere. Maybe I would not make a good mother, which is why motherhood was being withheld from me. Maybe I would have children and then regret it later. Maybe this was not a fair ask. Daily, I had to fight and wrestle with deep-seated insecurities to convince myself that it was *perfectly fine* to want motherhood. The tipping point came when the miscarriages occurred. It would have been natural to expect the two miscarriages to make me feel even more diffident about motherhood. But what they did was the opposite; they legitimized my ambition. These two episodes, however ephemerally, showed me that the family I was dreaming of could be mine. There was nothing wrong or invalid or excessive about my desires and there was no need to intellectualize them or to prove my merit. This keyhole into the future became the source of light that illuminated the rest of my journey in the dark.

~

I dived back into the world of office work with presentations and spreadsheets, weekly status reports and calls. One of the big tasks awaiting me in the pipeline was conduction of in-house workshops on documentation. Our teams partnered with government schools to improve the quality of education in disadvantaged districts across the country, and it was imperative that we captured their engagement. So, in the months after the miscarriage, a colleague and I travelled to four locations in south India and conducted three-day documentation workshops.

I enjoyed the travel and interaction with diverse sets of people, even though fear of public speaking ensured that I had diarrhoea every morning before a session and shed an alarming amount of hair. When I returned at the end of the south Indian sojourn to Bangalore, I was dreaming of convalescence. But my manager dropped a bombshell. 'We are short of people. Can you do one workshop in the north as well?' She offered me a choice between Rajasthan and Uttarakhand. I picked the latter, having heard a lot about its scenic beauty from other travelling colleagues. Besides, I had already been to Rajasthan as a child and didn't fancy going into the searing heat of a desert in April. So, in a week's time, I flew to Dehradun, and from there my colleague Sahil and I set out on a six-hour car journey to Uttarkashi, our workshop destination.

Uttarkashi is a quaint little town nestled in the Himalayan mountain ranges. It is home to the Gangotri, one among the four Chota Char Dham pilgrimage sites. The Ganga winds its way in and out of the town and the place is dotted with temples, infusing the air with a sense of sacredness. Less than a year ago, Uttarakhand had been devastated by floods and landslides. A cloudburst had unleashed havoc, leading to the collapse of bridges and roads, destruction of buildings and the death and displacement of thousands. When I visited Uttarakhand, almost ten months later, the landscape still bore signs of the destruction. Roads had been washed away and construction debris was spattered across the countryside. We had to take an alternative, longer route between Dehradun and Uttarkashi; the regular road was closed for repairs.

Over the next few days in Uttarkashi, we went through the same old drill. Sahil and I unpacked our slides, set up shop and put out the same performance. By now we were a travelling workshop company. We handed out writing exercises and moderated group discussions in a crammed

hall with participants sitting on the floor and taking notes on
writing pads and laptops. Even though my limited Hindi came
in the way, the workshop progressed smoothly. On the last
day, Sahil and I wound up early and began the return journey
to Dehradun. We had a flight to catch at dawn for Bangalore.

During the onward journey to Uttarkashi, I had been
anxious about the work at hand. Even though we had
delivered the same workshop in four other locations prior
to this, every new audience posed a challenge. I was not in
the shape of mind to observe and appreciate the beauty of the
hills. But now, having completed all five workshops across the
country, I felt relaxed. I could gaze out of the window of our
vehicle and take in the vast and rugged landscape that rose on
either side.

The sun was setting and the air was beginning to get
chilly, but it was not cold yet. There was a slight drizzle. Tiny
makeshift stalls on the way sold tea and hot cups of instant
Maggi noodles. Maggi was a favourite in these parts where
resources were scarce, and instant noodles made for a quick
and hot meal. Our driver played melodies from ancient Hindi
films, one after the other, offering the perfect background
score for our journey. It was a serene and magical evening. It
was the kind of evening that didn't come often—a reward for
my many days of toil and unrest. And now that it was there
I closed my eyes and held it close to my chest. All battles had
been laid to rest. All victories and defeats tallied. Everything
was in its place and life was unfolding as it should.

Sahil tapped my shoulder and said, 'Look.' In that
millisecond I wondered what could possibly be there to see
specifically on this lonely road. I looked out of the window
on his side and saw the most magnificent rainbow I had ever

seen in my life splashed across the sky. A colourful arc painted on a blue-and-white canvas stretching from one end of the horizon to the other. We stopped and got out of the car to admire the rainbow and take some pictures on our phones.

I have already spoken about the lingo unique to fertility forums on the Internet. There is shorthand for all the jargon that encompasses ART and euphemisms to smoothen the rough edges of pain and loss. The terms 'angel baby' and 'rainbow baby' belong to this idiom. Babies lost to miscarriage are referred to as 'angel babies', and the baby born after a miscarriage is called a 'rainbow baby'. I had lost two children to miscarriage and was still recovering from the last loss. I was waiting to complete the workshops and submit myself to the rigours of yet another IVF cycle. The timing of the rainbow couldn't have been more apt. It felt as if life was reaching out to me in some way, revealing itself a tiny bit, unravelling a fragment of its unfathomable mysteries. Life was saying the storm is passing and there is a rainbow around the bend. The heaviness will dissipate. Hold on. Just a little longer.

18

How Much Is Too Much?

On 11 April 2014, Archana was admitted to a birthing clinic in Calicut. By then she had gone past forty weeks. Doctors induced labour in the morning, but even after twelve hours she was dilated by only 2 cm. Her gynaecologist decided to perform a C-section.

At around eight that night I got a call from Gopal. The phone just stopped short of spontaneously combusting from the crackling happiness on the other end. He had a baby girl. I congratulated him and tried my level best to reciprocate the joy spilling over from his side.

A few minutes later, while having dinner, my phone beeped. The first photos of the baby were out. Frankly, newborns in the first days after birth look quite unappealing. They are too tiny to hold comfortably without being swaddled in layers of cloth. Their skin is wrinkled, they have little hair, and they keep their eyes shut. But Gayathri was an exception. I was told that when the nurse handed her to Gopal and Archana's parents, she had the air of a celebrity stepping off an aircraft and waving to a crowd of excited fans, fully ready and expecting the reception. She was the bright red colour of tomatoes, her cherubic face was framed by thick black hair, her eyes were open, and she smiled a coy smile. The video of that smile became a viral hit in our family.

The mood in my apartment in Bangalore was sombre. It had been a dreary Friday at work. I had spent all my time locked in a meeting room by myself and staring intently at the laptop, reliving the last miscarriage over and over again. Something unnameable—a concoction of sorrow, envy and guilt—churned inside and stopped me from feeling at peace. When I got the news about Gopal's baby, the heaviness became worse. I messaged my friend Sara for some consolation. She said bluntly, 'Don't wallow in self-pity.' I thought, 'You don't understand.' Ranjith and I went to the Mall that night, picked a movie at random and wordlessly surrendered ourselves to its universe. Did it work? Yes. To a certain degree. But then, how much pain can you swap for a movie outing?

~

In February 2014, two months prior to the Uttarakhand trip, I had gone back to the IVF clinic to start another FET cycle with the two embryos left in the freezer. Dr Leela began the FET regimen by monitoring the thickness of my endometrium; a thickness of 8 mm or above is considered desirable. Until then, achieving that thickness had not been a headache, but this time my uterine lining refused to cooperate, staying way below the required mark.

One of the probable causes for a thin endometrium is poor oestrogen levels. But I was already on estradiol valerate, taking nine tablets a day to boost the production of oestrogen. This was the maximum dose possible. My Google research told me that another cause for a poor endometrium was uterine surgery. There was a likelihood that the D&C done five months ago may have damaged my uterine lining. But there was nothing that could be done now to undo the injury, if any.

Even by day fourteen of the cycle, endometrial thickness was only 7 mm, which was the cut-off value. Anything below that is considered suboptimal for transfer and is associated with reduced pregnancy chances. At exactly 7 mm, we were balancing on a tightrope, one foot in front of the other. Dr Leela took a tough call and decided to cancel the cycle. We had two precious embryos left and it didn't seem worthwhile to transfer them into a uterus that was acting so pricey.

I agreed with her. But what were we going to do differently the next time that would improve the endometrial lining? Were we just going to throw a coin in the air and hope that it is heads the second time? Fortunately, Dr Leela had a more concrete plan. This was one of the things I liked about her. She seemed to have a fix for every malady, never giving me the feeling that I had reached a dead end. She was like a street-side magician with many tricks in her bag, and if this one didn't work then she would pull out another. This was also one of the reasons why we never considered changing the clinic or doctor despite the many failed cycles.

Beneath her almost brusque terseness was a layer of genuine concern for the patient. It was a layer she didn't reveal very often. After the second miscarriage, when I sat in her room sobbing into my dupatta, she said, 'I didn't expect this to happen. I came happily to the clinic today hoping to see your baby on the ultrasound.'

She was always accommodative of my schedule as a working woman and mindful of the high costs of the treatment, waiving fees wherever possible. But most importantly, she did not apportion blame or responsibility for any failure to me, the patient, as doctors do sometimes, knowingly or unknowingly. It is easy to guilt-trip an IVF patient into believing that *she* is responsible for any lack of success. But Dr Leela always insisted on maintaining an objective, non-judgemental and scientific gaze on our infertility.

For the next attempt she suggested we try an experimental method involving Granulocyte Colony Stimulating Factor (G-CSF).

'G-CSF is a protein that can stimulate the growth of cells in the endometrium. We will directly inject it into the uterus a few days prior to the transfer,' explained Dr Leela.

At the sound of G-CSF, my wilting hopes blossomed again. I was fascinated with new-fangled techniques and innovations in ART and eager to participate in the trials.

'Sure. Let's try that,' I jumped. My inner voice told me G-CSF was going to be the antidote to my endometrial blues.

Even though every failure felt like falling off a cliff we had climbed so painfully, these slight adjustments to treatment protocol gave us hope. With every cycle there was something narrowly new, some very tenuous straw to grasp, that gave us reason to feel the outcome was going to be different this time; that this particular drug or procedure or lifestyle alteration was going to make *all* the difference.

~

A week after I returned from Uttarakhand in end-April 2014, my period came visiting. Even after years of treatment, I harboured a secret wish for conception to happen on its own. Each time we had intercourse there was a small spike of excitement inside. Was this it? Would this be the time? When I heard stories of women who conceived naturally after a failed cycle, I took heart from them, willing the universe to give me the same lucky ending. In between the months of treatment, I continued to monitor ovulation and hoped that I was perhaps pregnant when my period skipped a day or two in coming. The social conditioning was so deep and ingrained, and the shame and stigma of treatment so heartfelt, that even while believing IVF was the answer to our infertility I wished it *wasn't* the answer. With the first cramping in my abdomen, the unmistakable warning signal of my period, the same disappointment and despair welled up inside. There was going to be no exemption. It would have to be IVF.

The next day I went to the clinic to begin the last of my FET exploits. I was mentally rigged to embark on another round of IVF stimulation if this FET cycle didn't result in a baby. Having come so far, I did not want to give up without using all our chances. It's recommended that couples plan for at least three to four IVF cycles, since the likelihood of achieving a live birth is highest at this point. I had gone through only two full cycles so far. So there were a few darts left to throw at the board.

Thinking along these lines would help me tone down my expectations from the current FET cycle and manage my panic if it didn't work. But my contingency planning didn't stop at that. What if this *and* the third IVF cycle (and all its adjunct FETs) didn't result in a baby? What would I do then? The mathematics suggested that at least some of us, despite our persistence, would never hit the mark. Should I keep on trying? How many more cycles should I inflict on myself? How much is too much?

Before we started IVF, Ranjith and I had promised each other to stick it out for three cycles, assuming it wouldn't take so long. But after all the failed attempts and two miscarriages we knew that it could potentially take much longer or maybe never happen. Before starting the current FET cycle, I asked Ranjith how much further we could go. Should we start thinking beyond three cycles?

We were sitting in the balcony sipping tea. We had a few minutes of quiet before the home engine was kickstarted.

'I don't know. There is no right or wrong answer to this.'

'I know that. But what do you think?'

'I would think we should stop at three. Especially given the long-term health risks attached to the process. You know that IVF has been linked to increased risk of ovarian cancer.'[1]

'Hmm.'

---

[1] The latest studies have indicated that there is no statistically valid direct correlation between the two. However, infertility itself is considered to be a risk factor for ovarian and other gynaecological cancers. The risk is slightly higher in women who have been treated with fertility drugs but have not had a live birth. (Source: I. Rizzuto, R.F. Behrens, and L. Smith, 'Is There an Increased Risk of Ovarian Cancer in Women Treated with Drugs for Subfertility?' Cochrane, June 2019, https://www.cochrane.org/CD008215/GYNAECA_there-increased-risk-ovarian-cancer-women-treated-drugs-subfertility#:~:text=The%20slight%20increase%20in%20ovarian,significant%20(%20P%20%3D%200.18.)

'But, and I know I am not right in saying this, if at the end of three cycles we still feel there is a good chance that it might happen with more attempts, we should keep trying.'

'But . . .'

'But the decision is yours. I am only saying this because you asked me. I don't want to push you any further than you have already gone.'

'Why does the buck always stop with me? Why do I have to take all the decisions?'

'Please, let's not get started on this. I am with you on this. If we stop at three, that's fine. If we decide to go beyond three, that's fine as well. Let's check with Dr Leela as well what she thinks.'

On my part, I was at risk of suffering from an unhealthy obsession. With IVF, I had hope. Without IVF, I had nothing. So despite all the hardships of treatment, it was tempting to keep on trying. It was easy to think that the next turn would bring a change of luck. But there is a line that separates determination from self-destruction, and with IVF that line was dissolving. On most days of the month, I felt happy, confident, successful and in control of my life and destiny. But when a new cycle of treatment started, the job, home, friends, family, marriage . . . everything dematerialized, faded away, became indistinct. Only the concrete, substantive absence of a child remained.

The worst was when a cycle worked and I got pregnant. For the weeks the pregnancy lasted, I cut myself off from the beats of everyday life, directing all my energies towards keeping the pregnancy safe. And when a pregnancy progressed as far as it did the last time and *then* failed, I was ruined. When I woke up the day after my last miscarriage, it felt like I had been sleeping for weeks and the whole world had marched ahead while I was forgotten and left behind. Everything in the never-ceasing cycles of nature had carried on as usual—some flowers bloomed, some withered, some trees shed their leaves persuaded by the October breeze, some stood their ground, some babies were birthed, some died. Only I was frozen in a globule of time staring at the rush and flow of mortal life outside. It took me a long time to step out and start walking with the others. So I promised myself, three IVF cycles and no more. After that I would have to walk away in the interest of keeping the compartments of my heart and brain intact.

~

There was some unexpected good news at the IVF clinic. Sini was back at work after having her baby. A relative had offered to come from Kerala to look after her three-month-old son while she resumed duties at the hospital. Seeing her face in the clinic was a shot of serotonin for me. My mood perked up.

My endometrial lining got off to another slow start, reaching only 6.7 mm on day ten. On day eleven, G-CSF was introduced in a procedure that resembled IUI. We would do an ultrasound two days later to check if it had worked. We were targeting a growth of at least 2 mm; then we could transfer the embryos with some degree of confidence. On day thirteen I went back to the clinic to review the thickness. When the ultrasound report came, my eyes popped out of their sockets. The endometrium had grown by 0.2 mm—by two decimal points. *Is this what G-CSF amounted to?*

Dr Leela was not surprised. She went through the report and said, 'Well, it hasn't worked for anyone!', making me feel like a complete idiot for placing so much faith in G-CSF. It was an experimental procedure that had failed all others; Dr Leela had seen no harm in trying it on one more guinea pig.

We waited three more days to see if there could be a late response. On day sixteen, the endometrial thickness was 7.1 mm. Only 0.1 mm better than during my cancelled cycle in February. This was a cruel joke. So much for believing that G-CSF would expand my endometrium into a fifteen-inch foam mattress!

Dr Leela came to the ultrasound monitor to examine the endometrium with her own set of eyes. She decided there was no point in postponing embryo transfer indefinitely, waiting for the perfect conditions. Yes, my chances were reduced because of a thin endometrial lining, but I certainly had no chance of getting pregnant while the embryos resided in cold storage. Better to put them inside my uterus and see if they would thrive. On the upside, even though the lining was only 7 mm thick, the endometrial pattern was promising. It was a triple lining endometrium containing a light line in the middle surrounded by two dark lines. Some studies have shown that a trilaminar pattern is correlated with higher implantation and pregnancy rates. Well, something is better than nothing.

On the day of the embryo transfer, Praveen defrosted the two remaining day-three eight-cell embryos. By now they had been in the lab for more than a year. I lay on the bed in the operating room with a sheet pulled over my half-naked body, waiting for the procedure to begin. Dr Leela first went into the IVF lab where Praveen had placed the embryos under a microscope for her. The lab was adjacent to the operating theatre where the transfer took place. From my bed I could see Dr Leela peering into the microscope. When she walked into the operating theatre she appeared unhappy. She pulled on a pair of gloves and went about her job, mentioning almost in passing that one of the embryos had not survived the thawing process.

Her words wiped out my remaining optimism like a broom going over a cobweb. Now there was only one embryo to drop on a uterine lining that was only 7 mm. With grade-A day-five blastocysts and a uterine lining that peaked at 10 mm, I had just about scraped through to get pregnant. What were my chances in such a depleted scenario? I doubted if we should even go through with the charade of an embryo transfer.

Perhaps seeing my visible disappointment, Dr Preetha butted in encouragingly. 'All our single-embryo transfers at the clinic have been successful. I am sure this will work too.'

If that was the case, why hadn't we opted for a single-embryo transfer (SET) earlier? SETs at the clinic had been successful before, but there was no evidence to suggest that *because* this was a SET it would work. Dr Leela didn't share her enthusiasm either and seemed slightly irritated by this false correlation.

Praveen brought the lone embryo in a catheter from the lab and handed it to Dr Leela. She pushed it inside my vagina, watching the blob[2] tumble down the narrow passage to my uterus on an ultrasound monitor. As it happened every time, the crowd in the room urged me to look at the screen and take heart from knowing that the seed had been

---

[2] The blob on the screen was not the eight-cell embryo, which is invisible to the naked eye. It was an air bubble inserted along with the embryo so that its path was traceable.

planted. Acquiescing, I tried to drum up feeling for the moment, but felt nothing, drained by the series of mishaps of the IVF cycle. My morale was resting firmly somewhere near rock bottom.

Soon the room emptied out and I was left alone to run down the clock till I could have use of my feet again. There was a forty-five-minute resting period in the operating theatre before being shifted to the recovery room. This period was meant to give the embryos some quiet settling-down time in their new territory. Sini waltzed in and out to check on me. But an uncomfortably cold room and a too-full bladder (required for ultrasound imaging) were making me edgy. Lying still on the hospital bed, chained to absolute passivity, holding back the urine was an impossible feat.

During my first transfer, Dr Leela had offered to drain the urine using a urinary catheter. Subsequently, fearing the risk of infection, she refused and insisted that I wait at least an hour before relieving myself. I would distract myself by chatting with Sini. This time I had gone overboard. Fearing that my bladder might not be full enough, I had gulped down at least two litres of water. After half an hour it became impossible to think about anything other than peeing.

Sini tried all sorts of diversionary tactics but I felt I was close to soiling the bed and my dignity. I asked her desperately, 'Can I go to the restroom?'

'Not yet. You have to wait for another fifteen minutes.'

I didn't think I would make it that far.

'Do you want a bedpan?' she suggested.

I thought for a second. I had never used one before, but desperate times needed desperate measures.

'OK. I will take it.'

I lifted my derriere off the bed, resting my body weight on my elbows and shoved the steel basin underneath. Making sure I had positioned it accurately, I let go. For the first time in my adult life I achieved the gravity-defying and precision-demanding task of peeing into a basin while being flat-out horizontal. Sini stood at the door and looked away. Oh yes, it was very dignified.

~

It was May and pre-monsoon showers had begun. There was a light rain outside as I came home in the afternoon and set myself up for another two-week wait with Manu Joseph's brilliantly titled *The Illicit Happiness of Other People*. This time Ranjith and I occupied the guest bedroom because our own room carried the aura of previous failures. Moving out, I felt, helped to exorcise the scents, images and energy that emanated from those memories. We were going to make a fresh start in a novel setting, if only on the other side of the same block of concrete.

I also decided to rejig my approach to the two-week wait, replacing worry and paranoia with indulgence and celebration. I applied for leave for the whole two weeks and committed myself to a grand vacation within the four walls of my apartment. The number one rule of this holiday was I would do *only* the things that made *me* happy. Thus began a carefully planned routine of absolute do-nothingness: taking long naps in the middle of the day, watching pirated CDs of Malayalam films on my laptop, and overdosing on Bollywood trivia and gossip on my phone. The second rule was that I would eat heartily but make sure my food is healthy. So, no caffeine, no sugar, lots of fruit and vegetables with every meal and a dry fruit smoothie once a day. The third rule was that I wouldn't worry about anything. Well, that rule got broken a few times every day, but I followed the first two stringently. I gave in to my cravings without feeling any pangs of guilt. My skin glowed and I gained a couple of kilos. The sparkle was back in my thirty-two-year-old eyes. Having only one embryo also meant that the pressure was off. If nothing else, I had been able to prise some leisure out of an IVF cycle. *Why hadn't I thought of this before?*

19

Take Nothing for Granted

I missed the naming ceremony of Gopal's baby girl because I was in the middle of the IVF cycle. I would have missed it anyway. I did not wish to face the entire family on an occasion that celebrated something I was yet to accomplish. Just visualizing everyone's sympathetic eyes and unspoken questions for Ranjith and me was enough to make that decision. To make up for our absence, Ranjith and I visited Gopal and Archana in Calicut a few days before the ceremony and dropped off gifts for the baby. If Gopal and Archana were hurt by my actions they didn't say so. They were perhaps too busy and sleep-deprived to notice. But I was concerned that Amma would not let me get away with this meanness. I thought she would insist that I set aside my ego and join the ceremony. After all, I had only one brother and it was his first child. After all, this occasion was not about me, it was about Gopal and Archana. But on the day of the event, when someone asked why I had not come, Amma brushed off the question saying, 'She was here a few days ago. How many visits can be made in a week?' When I heard that, I was so grateful for her ability to shut people up when needed, for backing me in front of others. But even I knew what she *actually* thought about my absence—that it was petty and small-minded.

~

The beta hCG test was scheduled for a Thursday. I decided to do some advance testing at home on Tuesday. No matter how many times I had been thrown off by HPTs, I still persisted with them. But until Monday night there was not a single pregnancy symptom. Since I had been pregnant twice before, there was physical memory to serve as reference, but no tic or twitch presented itself to be decoded as a sign of pregnancy. I would have gladly written away our apartment, cars and other savings to feel the faintest flash of giddiness, fatigue or nausea, but that night, as I watched an angry rain lash the city from the balcony of our sixth-floor apartment, I felt as un-pregnant as ever. My fifteen-day vacation was coming to an end.

A pregnancy symptom is, however, a fickle and deceptive mistress. When the symptoms are in full bloom the test may show nothing. When there is no trace of any symptom the test can throw up a surprise. The next day I did the HPT. After fortifying myself to see a single line, I dropped two droplets of urine in the test area and waited. The first and then the second pink line appeared promptly. I was surprised and happy but not fully trusting. The HPT was repeated the next day and the day after that. The second pink line continued to manifest.

On Thursday, I went to the clinic for the beta hCG test. By twelve I got a call from Dr Preetha. The value was 605 mIU/ml! I was expecting a number in the 200–300 range, so this toppled my highest estimates. I was happy, but it was still not time to celebrate. The value had to multiply. On Saturday, the results of the repeat beta hCG came in. The value was 1230 mIU/ml! It had doubled, more than doubled. When I heard that number over the phone, the pregnancy finally became doubtless and trustworthy. I went to the small puja alcove in our home, folded my hands, closed my eyes and burst into the happiest tears I have ever cried.

After the positive beta hCG test, a few symptoms crept up. There was nausea from a heightened sense of smell. I could not tolerate lying down on the living room sofa because the fabric smelled of everything I had ever eaten sitting on it. I made an urgent appointment for sofa shampooing. When I took a break from healthy eating and ordered pizza, I regretted the decision almost immediately. The sharp odour of garlic bread that came with it was too overpowering for my sensitive nostrils. The smells on the streets we are normally inured to— of cow dung, open drains, garbage cans—made me choke, but I stopped short of vomiting.

Morning sickness is believed to be a sign of a healthy, viable pregnancy. Studies have shown that women who have both nausea *and* vomiting are much less likely to have a miscarriage. So I was grateful for the nausea but wished it extended to vomiting too. I longed to throw up my meals, as proof of a thriving pregnancy, but sadly never came that far. Even the signs that existed were inconsistent. Sometimes I felt giddy if I went a couple of hours without eating anything. At other times I didn't feel hungry at all from afternoon to midnight. I stood in front of the bathroom mirror daily and examined my breasts and abdomen, looking for some evidence of the life growing inside, but it was too early for any such clues. There was very little physical manifestation of the pregnancy. It made me want to fast forward to the stage when the pregnancy displayed itself in a rotund, protruding belly and I didn't have to keep answering the question in my head, 'Am I *really* pregnant? Have I *stopped* being pregnant since the last time I felt giddy or sick?'

The general mood in our house and family was one of cautious optimism. For the first time we felt secure enough to share the news with immediate family (beyond my mother): Ranjith's parents, his sister and my brother. This was the best start to a pregnancy so far and Ranjith was convinced that we were finally closing the doors on infertility. I shared his confidence to a large extent because the beta hCG values looked so promising. We both waited eagerly for the first ultrasound, two weeks away.

~

It was a Sunday afternoon. The pregnancy seemed safely and firmly perched on the back of strong beta hCG numbers. With just a week to go for the first ultrasound, my miscarriage radar was lowered. The house help was on leave and the kitchen sink was submerged under a pile of dirty dishes.

'Shall we go out for lunch? We can go to that north Karnataka place,' Ranjith suggested.

'Isn't that too far? It's forty-five minutes away. I am not sure if such a long car ride is OK to do now.'

'What's wrong with you? There is no need to place ourselves under house arrest to protect this pregnancy. Eating at a restaurant has not been known to cause miscarriage. Please stop thinking like this.'

Ranjith was beginning to get impatient with my timidity.

He was right. Acceding to his superior reasoning, I got
dressed, feeling mildly thrilled at the prospect of airing my
new kurta and silver earrings. There was some weight gain
from three weeks of staycation, but I could still fit comfortably
into my existing wardrobe.

It was a vegetarian restaurant in Kormangala that offered
plantain-leaf meals, hot jowar rotis topped with cubes of
butter and accompanied by a variety of curries, chutneys and
deep-fried snacks. The dishes were flung on plantain leaves
by overenthusiastic servers in an unremitting stream. It was
left to the diners to keep up or keep out. We sat down at one
of the last tables still available, a four-seater in the centre
of the first-floor dining hall, and waited for the service to
start. While the plantain leaves were being distributed, my
bladder beckoned and I got up to address it before the meal
marathon began.

The bathroom was located one level below; I opened the
door and peered inside gingerly. It was too wet for my liking,
but not obviously dirty. Closing the door behind me, I undid
the knot of my salwar and sat on the commode when my eyes
fell on my panties. I went cold. There was a splash of blood.
Dark red, almost brown, blood, as if someone had punched
me in the gut and I had started bleeding through my vagina.

My eyes stayed locked on the blood, arms and legs ice-
cold. The blood had come so unannounced, so unnoticed,
that even *my* imagination, my ever-vigilant, ever-suspicious
imagination, which foresaw dangers at every door, had not
contrived this scenario. After a few minutes I gathered myself
and went back upstairs to inform Ranjith, ready to pick up
my handbag and sprint out of the restaurant. *See, I was right.
Coming this far was a bad idea. I need to get back to the safety*

of my bedroom. But Ranjith stayed calm. He insisted we stay put, finish our meal and then drive back.

'I am sure this is nothing. Remember, we read that some spotting is common in pregnancy. Relax,' he said, turning to ask for refills of buttermilk.

It was surreal, forcing myself to sit down in that restaurant, trying to hold my splintering self together while believing that something fatal had happened or was about to happen to my baby. I chewed down one jowar roti and asked the dumbfounded server to clear the leaf while Ranjith polished off each course from roti to anna-saaru to mosaranna.

Hadn't he understood what I said? How could he be so unconcerned?

During the drive home, Ranjith reiterated that I was overreacting. I was deaf to his words, sitting cross-legged in the car, impatient to get home as quickly as possible. I had had only a brief glimpse of my blood-stained panties in the restaurant's dimly lit washroom and I was not sure if I had interpreted it correctly. Maybe it was an unwashed stain on the fabric. Maybe it was just discoloured vaginal discharge. Maybe it was a phantom image created by my brain as a result of extreme paranoia. I kept my hopes alive, attributing alternative meanings to the stain.

When we arrived home I dashed to the bathroom and checked again. The blood was still there, it hadn't miraculously vanished in the previous one hour. I touched it with my finger and brought the finger to my nose. It had the salty, tangy smell of blood. This was no spectre of my overwrought imagination, this was as fresh and tactile as knife-cutting-finger blood. I came out, threw myself on the bed in the guest room and cried my eyes out. Ranjith sat next to me and tried to say that everything would be OK, but I was not falling for the platitudes again.

After an hour, when I had recovered from the tears, I went to the kitchen and made myself a cup of tea. I huddled on the diwan, cradling the mug of hot liquid in my hands and took stock of the wreckage. It was a Sunday so there would be no doctors available at the IVF clinic. We would have to go to the main hospital, and our previous experience in that facility was hardly encouraging. Besides, I was only six weeks pregnant. Six weeks is the earliest anything can be seen via an ultrasound, so if we went now there was a good chance that the ultrasound would be inconclusive. And if we did do an ultrasound and saw nothing it would just add to the scare. I felt it was better to wait two more days before heading to the IVF clinic. That would give more time for the foetus to grow and thereby result in a more definitive ultrasound. Waiting two more days also meant the ultrasound would be done on a Tuesday. Tuesday was my lucky day because I was born on a Tuesday and the first positive HPT had been done on a Tuesday. I believed if I went on Tuesday the miscarriage could be averted. But this meant I would have to last the next forty-eight hours in a suspended state. Forty-eight hours in a state of tense darkness, not knowing if the bleeding indicated a miscarriage or a harmless occurrence common to pregnancy.

The pros and cons were balanced on my mental weighing scale until eventually superstition outweighed all other considerations. I was a big believer in lucky days and signs of things to come and didn't want to jeopardize this pregnancy by going to the hospital on the wrong day of the week. So I made the decision to wait and articulated my reasons to Ranjith. He nodded in agreement. Even he knew that if this pregnancy was falling through, then waiting a couple of days was not going to alter its fate.

For the next two days the spotting continued on and off, but there was no pain or contraction. I tried to stay off my feet and googled tirelessly to find an explanation for the bleeding but could not find a search result that suggested it was going to be all right. Every time I went to the bathroom and saw the discharge in my panties, I came undone, imploding inside like a child's teetering tower of wooden blocks. *Was this one going to fail too? Three back-to-back? Weren't the doubling beta hCG values supposed to mean something? Could I take nothing for granted?*

~

On Tuesday, at the IVF clinic, I sought to downplay the bleeding, not even using the word 'blood' while reporting it. I wanted to break it gently to Dr Preetha and others, being more concerned about *their* disappointment at my consecutive failures, like that student who can't ace an examination despite the best efforts of the teacher.

Dr Preetha expressed surprise at seeing me one week prior to the date the ultrasound was due.

'I saw some brown discharge on my panties and thought it would be best to double check with you guys,' I said casually, but I was fooling no one.

She picked up the phone, called the radiologist and said, 'I have a patient here who is six weeks pregnant and has bleeding. I am sending her for a TVS immediately.'

The pregnancy was faring much better than I thought. The ultrasound showed that at six weeks, two days there was a single live intrauterine pregnancy. The foetal heart rate was 103 bpm. The bleeding was due to a subchorionic collection around the gestational sac. A subchorionic bleed[1] is usually harmless and resolves on its own. All the foetal parameters were within range and there was no reason to suspect another miscarriage.

I met Dr Leela after the ultrasound and she made a couple of changes to the prescription to keep the bleeding in check. She discontinued a vaginal suppository and replaced it with an oil-based intramuscular injection on my request. I worried that my nail might irritate vaginal tissue and provoke further bleeding while inserting the pill. Besides, the suppository was a messy affair, causing white, chalky discharge. Every time I felt a release of the discharge, my heart skipped a beat. Was it blood or just the suppository? But the injection meant I had to visit the clinic on alternate days. I was all right with this too because it gave me a reason to get out of the house even if it took me only so far as the clinic. I could have ten minutes of confidence-boosting and heart-reassuring conversation with Sini.

The consultation over, I gathered the unwieldy hospital file and took the elevator to the parking lot. By now my heart was light as a feather. There was a non-ominous explanation for the blood. The pills and injections had been rearranged

---

[1] 'A subchorionic bleed (also known as a subchorionic hematoma) is the accumulation of blood between the uterine lining and the chorion (the outer fetal membrane, next to the uterus) or under the placenta itself.' (Source: Catherine Donaldson-Evans, 'Subchorionic Bleeding during Pregnancy', *What To Expect*. Reviewed 28 October 2019, https://www.whattoexpect.com/pregnancy/pregnancy-health/complications/subchorionic-bleeding.aspx.)

to suit my convenience and the danger needle was back to its resting position. The only annoying thing was Ranjith's smug 'I-told-you-so' expression. I hated his unflappable calm and perpetual optimism. It made me look crazy next to him, but it was his turn to gloat.

On the drive back I called my mother and Ranjith's mother to provide an after-the-fact report. Ranjith felt it was best to be transparent about the highs and lows of the pregnancy. I didn't agree with him entirely, and their reaction was exactly what I had anticipated: panic. I was asked to immobilize myself. Hire full-time help. If that was not feasible, they offered to come and take care of me while I took bed rest, getting up only for bathroom breaks. They quoted from the protocol of *other* IVF clinics.

'Here it's the norm for IVF centres to dictate nine months of strict bed rest for the woman. Some clinics require hospitalization for the full term. What on earth is your doctor up to?' Amma said, incensed.

They were horrified that Dr Leela was so irresponsible as to suggest that I carry on with my day-to-day activities, which surely had led to the bleeding in the first place. They were especially concerned because they believed this was an 'artificial' pregnancy and that too at an advanced age, therefore warranting extra care and precaution. I tried telling them that this connection between bed rest and success of an IVF pregnancy was misplaced. But who was listening?

As far as I know, there is very little a woman can do to sabotage her pregnancy. The most common cause of a first-trimester miscarriage is chromosomal abnormalities, and bed rest cannot reverse a genetic defect. Even though miscarriage rates are higher in IVF pregnancies (this may be because IVF is attempted by those at an advanced maternal age or having pre-existing medical conditions) studies have not been able to suggest that bed rest or lack of bed rest is a factor. Yes, maternal trauma is a factor, but walking, cooking or going to a theatre to watch a movie do not constitute maternal trauma. Yes, advanced maternal age also poses a risk, but that cannot be undone by physical immobility. Moreover, I was only thirty-two, and in fertility medicine thirty-five years or older is typically considered advanced maternal age. And what about 'artificial'? Well, technology is embedded in most modern-day enterprises from food to education to interpersonal relationships. Why assume a discriminatory stance only towards conception?

The notion of 'artificiality' or 'inauthenticity' may have something to do with the label 'test-tube baby' and the alienating image of a newborn lying curled up inside a test tube, which is used to advertise fertility clinics. IVF does not involve culturing babies inside a test-tube. An embryo is placed in an IVF incubator for two to five days, a microscopic cluster of a few cells, before it is transferred to the woman's uterus. The most crucial element of conception— implantation—occurs inside the woman, and the baby grows drawing its nourishment from the woman's body. This cannot be replicated in a lab, at least not yet.

I managed to stave off unsolicited offers of help and continued to cook, clean, work on the computer and hang out at the Mall, to the utter dismay of my mother and in-laws.

The bleeding continued for the next seven days until the second ultrasound. Despite having a name and a benign explanation for it, every time I saw the blood on my underwear I got that hollow, sinking feeling. The feeling that I was skating on a thin sheet of ice that could crack open any instant, that there wasn't much to separate staying on the frost and falling off it. Every move had to be tentative.

~

A week later, at the second ultrasound, I was seven weeks and two days pregnant. Dr Sushma, the radiologist, dressed the transducer in a fresh condom, smeared gel on it and shoved it inside my vagina, her eyes shifting to study the images on the screen. A few minutes into the scan, she declared, 'Everything is normal.'

I went back to the waiting hall and studied the two-page report with the polaroid-like black-and white-photos of the foetus pinned to it. The foetal heart rate was a healthy 137 bpm. Tick. The subchorionic collection was present but it was not posing any problems. Tick. And the foetus . . . the foetus was not growing as expected.

The gestational age as per the ultrasound was only six weeks and four days—which was almost four days behind the dating by last menstrual period (seven weeks, two days). It is assumed that a foetus grows at the rate of 1 mm per day from six weeks onwards till nine and a half weeks. In the last scan, the crown rump length (CRL[2]) was 3.8 mm. If it had grown by 1 mm every day, then the CRL should have been 10.8 mm,

---

[2] Verywell Family, 'The baby is measured, in centimetres, from the top of their head (crown) to the bottom of their buttocks (rump).' (Source: Krissi Danielson, 'Crown Rump Length [CRL] on Ultrasounds', last updated on 2 February 2020, https://www.verywellfamily.com/crown-rump-length-crl-2371608.)

but it was only 6.8 mm. *What happened to the three days in between? Why hadn't the foetus grown as much?*

I took the report back to Dr Sushma who was in the middle of another scan. She finished the scan and stepped out. I told her about the missing three days of foetal growth.

'Oh that! No, the machine's margin of error is plus or minus six days. We are well within that range and there is no need for any concern.'

I was not satisfied. At seven weeks the average CRL of a normal foetus was 11 mm, while the CRL of my foetus was only 6.8 mm. A low CRL is associated with chromosomal anomalies, even if the heartbeat is normal. It could mean miscarriage or severe birth defects. In the last pregnancy I obsessed over the foetal heart rate; in this pregnancy it was the turn of CRL. I checked with Dr Leela and Dr Preetha. Both had the same explanation, but I was not convinced. As far as I was concerned there was something definitely wrong. As always, I didn't trust anyone who told me that everything was fine.

That night, to confirm my suspicions, I sought a second opinion by emailing a renowned IVF specialist in Mumbai. He was the creator of a massive corpus of online resources on infertility and offered a free consultation online. I was an avid consumer of his blog and trusted his judgement. In a few hours, he sent a cryptic response, 'Wait and watch.' I surmised from the non-committal reply that he too thought CRL was a concern because he did not offer any reassurance. This was perhaps understandable, given the data available, but I used it to feed my conspiracy theories.

The next day I trotted back to the clinic and begged Dr Leela to order another ultrasound.

She rolled her eyes. 'It doesn't help at this stage to do a scan every day and get frantic about the numbers.'

'Yes, but the foetus is not growing at the rate of 1 mm per day. Something has to be wrong.'

'No, the foetus does not always grow in such a precise, symmetrical manner. We must wait for a critical mass of time to elapse before deducing anything. If the next scan fifteen days later shows a gestational age of at least eight weeks, four days, there is no cause for concern,' she explained, drawing on her last reserves of patience.

I left the consultation room convinced that this pregnancy was going downhill and eventually everyone would come to the same conclusion and *I* would be proven right. I refused to believe the radiologist, I refused to believe Dr Leela. I believed Google. And according to Google this was a failing pregnancy, or one with severe abnormalities so we would have to abort sooner or later.

I was testing Ranjith's patience and commitment to the marriage every day with my half-baked theories from the Internet. Two days after the last consultation, at breakfast, I was in the middle of a lecture on how this pregnancy was going to fail, based on my superior understanding of reproductive science, when Ranjith decided enough was enough.

'I have no interest in this kind of pessimism and I would rather go by the doctor's words and believe that things are working well. If you want to drown in despair even before anything has gone wrong, that is your prerogative. But I don't want to be a party to this, and I certainly don't want to hear of it.'

I was stunned by the firmness in his voice. He rarely asserted himself so sternly. He was usually a silent spectator to my episodes of hyper-anxiety. I fell quiet. I took a step back. He hadn't said anything to disprove my conviction, but I thought, at least outwardly, to honour his wishes, I would stop being a messenger of gloom and doom. For a limited period of two weeks, I would pretend to be a positive-thinking, mature, emotionally stable person. How tough was that?

I am sure that not all women who go through IVF experience this level of fear and doubt. Maybe they don't want to know about the behind-the-scenes science or choose not to get tied up in knots over each medical detail. Maybe they are happy with a broad understanding of their condition and trust what the doctors have to say, leaving the rest to God or faith or destiny. Maybe they believe that if they are careful, positive or pious enough, everything will work out just fine. Maybe they believe in miracles. Ranjith himself is like that. But I was a born worrier, a born doubter, and IVF only served to amplify my anxiety to explosive levels. This book is mainly a documentation of the number of times and number of ways in which I fell apart.

I went back to working from home. Time continued to crawl, from one two-week segment to another. The few hours spent in front of the laptop offered respite from speculating about the pregnancy. Every other waking minute was spent reading the unreliable signals emitted by my body, browsing pregnancy forums and predicting the future of my unborn child. I heaved a tiny breath of relief for each night and day that went by without bleeding, without pain, without missing any of the pregnancy symptoms. And like this I inched towards the next ultrasound, grateful for each unremarkable day.

~

It was a Tuesday again. I was nine weeks and two days pregnant. If the ultrasound showed foetal growth corresponding to at least eight weeks and four days, we could conclude that the baby was fine. That was the best-case scenario, but I didn't expect such a straightforward result. I expected complications, more doubt and uncertainty. I went in fully rehearsed for another cliffhanger.

In the familiar dark ultrasound room, Dr Sushma's face was lit up by the light from the blurry images on the screen. She tapped the keys to minimize and maximize sections, noting down measurements on a piece of paper. A few minutes in, she declared again, 'Everything is normal.' I was unimpressed.

I got dressed and sat down beside Ranjith in the waiting area to personally scrutinize the report. The foetus stood at the gestational age of eight weeks and four days. Tick. The heart rate was 178 bpm. Tick. The subchorionic collection was gone. Tick. No anomalies were noted. Tick. Everything *was* normal. Tick. My mouth dropped open slightly. What? My hunch was wrong? Everything was *fine*?

I put the report down in disbelief and looked around the room, my heart swelling up, a smile tingling at the edges of my lips. After the bends and curves of the path so far, this seemed too straight, too easy, an anticlimax. It was like turning a corner inside a maze and, out of the blue, running into the exit. But what a relief and joy it was to have at last a simple, clear, unambiguously positive result. I held Ranjith's hands tightly and told him, 'Everything is fine.' His eyes glistened as he squeezed my hand back.

That was to be my last ultrasound at the IVF clinic. I left for home a little sad that I wouldn't be coming to the clinic any more. Three weeks later, at twelve weeks, four days, I went to the main hospital for the next ultrasound. I got the pink folder, heard the baby's heartbeat. I consulted Dr Leela at the general gynaecology OPD. I had crossed the first trimester. I was bona fide pregnant now.

~

On 16 January 2015, at thirty-eight weeks, four days, I was wheeled into the operating theatre for an elective C-section. The anaesthetist stood behind my head and Ranjith, in scrubs, sat beside me on a stool next to the bed. My mother, Ranjith's parents and his sister waited outside in the labour ward.

The attendants placed a half-screen at my chest to block my view so that I would not be terrified at the sight of a knife splitting open my stomach. Dr Leela walked in and the room swung into action. Before making the incision, she asked what I wanted, 'A boy or a girl?', as if this was made to order. I chose girl. Within a few minutes there was a cry, a short, sharp cry; it was the cry of someone who had been woken up by an annoying disturbance but quickly went back to sleep.

Dr Leela noted, with a twinge of disappointment, 'It's a boy.'

'It's OK. I am good with boys too.'

Tears had started running down my face, alarming the anaesthetist. 'Why are you crying? Are you in pain?'

I quickly smiled through my moist eyes and said, 'No, I am just happy.'

He patted my face and wiped my tears since both my hands were hooked to various instruments.

A nurse brought my baby wrapped in a green hospital sheet close to my face so that I could have a look and plant a kiss on him. My first thought was, 'Oh no! He has *my* nose!' Then the nurse took him away to check his vital signs, clean him up and place him in the neo-natal intensive care unit (NICU) for observation while Dr Leela and others sewed up my abdomen. Ranjith followed the baby into the NICU while I slipped into a welcome bout of sedation.

I don't think Ranjith and I exchanged any words in the five or ten minutes that it took to cut up my stomach and extricate the baby. What words were there to say?

Can any words, poetic or otherwise, communicate the mix of emotions that anchored us to that wordless moment when our child was born? I doubt it. It's a moment that stays locked up in the joint memory vault of our lives, like precious silver or crystal. We retrieve it occasionally, admire it and put it back. Embellishing it with words would only have ruined its shine.

20

Why Want Children?

I hated being a child. From as far back as I can remember, I had the bearing of an adult. It was harrowing to be trapped inside a child's body for years and years. I waited impatiently for adulthood to arrive and set me free.

As a teenager I dreaded young children. Baby talk made me cringe. Toddlers needed too much attention. Those who were five-years-plus could be tolerated for short intervals. With those who were ten years and older, I relaxed. Now we were on the same page, both of us wanted to be left alone.

As a young wife I hated how children hogged all the attention in a room. Especially when I had no children of my own to hog any attention.

Why then did I want children? It is the biggest contradiction of my infertility experience that I had no single, personal, unassailable answer to the question. I was a racehorse with blinkers on, eyeing only the finish line, blind to what rewards or trials awaited me after that. I had wholeheartedly bought into the myth of motherhood as the 'ultimate' source of meaning and fulfilment, and it was difficult to tell how much of my desire came from traditional norms and how much from the urge to raise and nurture a new person. It was part of my template for an 'ideal' life and I didn't want to deviate from it. Despite my conviction in the 'necessity' of having children, there was also a rankling worry about my unease around them. Did I really want children? Would I make a good-enough mother? I carried both in my heart, the dread and the desire. But I reckoned that once I had my *own* child, I would know what to do. When the time came, I would be ready.

~

My son, lying curled in my womb, must have giggled at that proclamation. Ready? Ready is what you are before stepping out for a dinner party. Ready is what you are when the Uber arrives. That word is highly inappropriate in the context of bringing up a child.

Things began smoothly enough. For the first forty days I had the following people to take care of Advaith: (listed in order of usefulness) my mother-in-law, my father-in-law, my mother, a full-time maid, a part-time maid, and a husband eager to earn his spurs as a father. I wondered why people made such a big fuss about child rearing. When I woke up on the forty-first day, the entire entourage had disappeared, except for my husband, who was at the bottom of the utility scale anyway. It took six months from then for me to be able to sleep lying down and one and a half years to make it through the night in that position. I researched extensively online on baby sleep and tried to implement every sleep training method, from Ferber to Tracy Hogg. Yet Advaith only napped for thirty minutes at a stretch, if at all, during the day, and this took at least thirty minutes of standing up and rocking him in my arms. At night he woke up anywhere between three and twenty times. Gopal, the more experienced parent, in a bid to pacify me, said, 'Don't worry. These months will go by in a blink.' I took his advice and blinked rapidly. Nothing changed. It was still 2 a.m. Advaith was awake and I was still rocking him.

By the time he turned eighteen months old, there was some respite. He was walking, sleeping for longer stretches and almost weaned off breast milk. I dropped nineteen kilos and two dress sizes. I resumed work, though part-time and only from home. I reclaimed my body and life to some extent.

Advaith too came into his own, expressing vehement dislike for some things and ardent love for others. He was transfixed by any device that rotated, from the drum of a concrete mixer to the blades of a kitchen blender. When we came to the page on ships and boats in his toddler book of vehicles, he turned the page impatiently. No wheels were a no-go. He had a white toy chest with a blue dolphin on it. It had a few toys but mostly books. Every meal time we picked three or four books and read animatedly about dancing giraffes, schoolgoing puppies and farting elephants. He lapped up any piece of information that his toddler brain could process: names of colours and shapes, numbers one to hundred, the alphabet, days of the week and months of the year. My mom-pride skyrocketed to unhealthy levels.

But having a two-year-old at home meant being a Bollywood back-up dancer, budding paediatrician and Michelin star chef, all in the same day. I forgot that bathrooms came with doors, learnt to answer questions intelligibly while brushing my teeth, and found it completely natural to throw a blanket over wetness and go back to sleep on the same bed. There were moments of bliss but they were separated by cycles of chaos. When he couldn't have what he wanted, Advaith would bang his forehead against the floor and yell non-stop. Onlookers must have presumed what a wicked mother I must be to elicit such a reaction from my son. He was petrified of crowds. When we went to Calicut for a wedding, I wore a toddler-accessory pinned to my saree all three hours of the function. Frankly, I started dreaming of playschool and crossed the days and months on the desk calendar to the time he would be eligible for it.

~

I have a photograph from Advaith's first day of school. It's a photograph I clicked with my eyes. He is wearing a yellow panda T-shirt paired with a black pair of jeans. A small cloth bag shaped like a robot is slung over his back. Inside there is a snack box filled with raisins and biscuits and a water bottle. He is skipping and hopping to the car, a radiant, spotless joy emanating from him. I stop midway and turned back to capture that frame; to memorialize that day in the album of his childhood. But if you look closely enough at that photograph, you will spot a grey cloud of worry tinging the otherwise immaculate sky, bearing the residual fears from my own first day of school.

At the age of four I went directly to a big formal school; there had been no preschool or playgroups to prepare for it. I was led into a large, dark hall and the doors were shut behind me. I thought I was never going to see my mother again. A bunch of us, tiny tots, sat in a circle, screaming our lungs out, hoping that the sound would penetrate the thick walls of this dungeon and reach the outside world. There were bright cut-out pictures pasted on the walls and teachers trying to pacify and distract us, but nothing could mitigate the terror and misery of the setting.

As Ranjith and I sat in the school director's room, I imagined that Advaith's unsuspecting happiness would be belied soon. There would be fierce protests, ear-rending cries, and our son would be scarred for life. The director finished her pep talk, got up and took Advaith by the hand to lead him inside.

'Just be cool. No extended farewells,' she warned.

We said a short, cheerful, 'Have a great day, Adu! Bye.'

I watched his face for any signs of crumpling.

He turned to us, simply said 'Bye' and walked inside without once looking back.

We waited outside the gates expecting to be called inside any minute for rescue. Ranjith was pacing up and down on the pavement outside. I waited in the car. Nothing happened.

After ninety minutes Advaith came out waving a piece of paper on which he had doodled with colour pencils.

'Amma, look what I did,' he said.

'Wow, did you do that yourself?'

After admiring his work of art, I checked his bag. The snack box was empty and the water bottle depleted. Ranjith and I probed him for a minute-by-minute account of school. But in the toddler world, what's past is past, even if it was only fifteen minutes ago. Aside of our lack of clarity on this point, Ranjith and I had the body language of cross-country runners who had just breasted the tape. We had made it.

Our son's first few days of school, though, were a little disorienting. To have the full range of my faculties and body parts all to myself felt a little strange. At home I could sit in a chair without fifteen kilograms of human flesh clambering all over me. I didn't have to fend off with one hand a visitor in the kitchen pulling out pots and pans out from the drawers while straining tea with the other. There was no intruder punching all the buttons on the washing machine while it was being loaded. I could do one thing at a time. How luxurious and extravagant!

I drop him off at the school gate every day, turn on my heels and start running back as if my life depended on it. Sometimes I forget that I came in a car. I don't linger in the school compound watching his back disappear indoors or start a conversation with the teacher on how he is doing. I can't risk losing a sliver of my already thin slice of solitary time.

But school offers only a four-hour blip in the day. There's still ten-odd hours of maniacal energy left to be harnessed on any given day. I invest in special-activity boxes, art and craft projects, a multitude of books. But it often feels as if the effort to execute a linear, sequential and productive activity with a preschooler is not worthwhile. My son has no faith in straight lines, a quick clean dash from point A to point B. He believes in squiggles and wiggles, waves and curls, all things that subvert the efficiency and boredom of straight lines. Left to himself he devises his own 'projects'. In fact, everything is a project.

Project I: Turn on every power switch in the house including those of the AC, microwave and washing machine. Step on the commode lid, climb on to the bathroom sink, reach for the power switch near the ceiling, turn on the geyser. Once you start a project, you must see it through.

Project II: Transport all the shoes from the shoe cabinet in the portico to the living room. Arrange them to spell 'ADVAITH' on the carpet. Project over.

Project III: Use a shovel from the beach toys kit to dig up some mud. Bring it to the kitchen, mix it with water and leaves, place it on a plate. Allow it to dry. Transfer it to the dining table, leaving behind a trail of mud and water. Pat yourself on the back for another project well executed.

Project IV: Identify the precise location of your mother's bladder by pulling up her T-shirt while she is lying on a bed reading a book. Fix your sight on it. Jump from a pillow and try to land on the target. Try, try again until you succeed.

Project V: Use sketch pens to make the white handwoven bedcover in the master bedroom more 'colourful' (his words, not mine).

There are some days when only fear of the Indian Penal Code and the crumbling infrastructure of Indian prisons has stopped me from acting on the murderous rage coursing through my veins. When I finish putting his Lego blocks back in their colour-coordinated boxes, he has pulled out the Scrabble board and letters. When I have just finished making dinner and am laying it on the table, he cracks open an unguarded egg on the kitchen counter, letting the yolk glaze the floor. It's a never-ending cycle of spin and tumble dry. And then I hark back to the good old days when I was childless. When I took afternoon naps, long baths, enjoyed movies in cinema halls and shopped carefree. What happened to those times, and what is the fuss about motherhood?

I know parents whose experience of infertility has made them immune to the hardships of parenting. They don't lose their cool or complain about the lack of free time. They are so grateful for this reward, made sweeter by the bitter pain of infertility. I am not one of them. Raising a child is relentlessly hard, and the long years I spent waiting for motherhood have not transformed me into an always-smiling, all-forgiving embodiment of patience and love. I am grateful for my son, but I do miss the spontaneity, ease and independence of my pre-motherhood days.

Some of it is because of how obsessive I am about nailing parenting and gifting my son the perfect childhood on a silver platter. This means protecting him from every harm, exposing him to diverse mental stimuli, and constructing an atmosphere of positive reinforcement and support. And in doing so I refuse to share responsibility with a grandparent or nanny. I take pride in being the world's foremost authority on Advaith, and the only person I would count as co-expert is Ranjith. But he has a busy full-time career that takes him out of town at least two days of the week, and his parenting philosophy doesn't even make for a full sentence. It amounts to 'let him be'. A minimal-thought and zero-interference approach. When our son is hungry, he will eat. When he is tired, he will sleep. And if he falls ill, he will recover.

As always, we are on two ends of the north–south axis. When I am tearing my hair out because my son has mixed up his home clothes, going-out clothes and bedtime clothes, or has missed his 4 p.m. snack or he has sneezed more than once, Ranjith barely registers an emotion. Like the coloured squares on a Rubik's cube, our ways are hard to align: My refusal to delegate. His inability to participate any further. My need for total control. His laissez faire mindset. But on nights that I lose sleep over imaginary fevers or play-date episodes I am convinced will damage my son for life, I look at my peacefully asleep husband and remind myself that it is absolutely imperative for a child who has a mother like me to have a father like him.

~

Before I had Advaith, I felt completely unqualified and ineligible for the job. Because of my general incompetence with children, I worried if I could bond with my child, if I would know how to play with, talk to and entertain him, if I was *enough* for him. But the last few years have proven my concerns supremely silly. My son is not a machine to learn to operate, or an instrument to learn to play. Loving and taking care of him has been intuitive and instinctive, as it is with any other human being. It required no special skill sets or talents or personality traits.

Besides, how difficult can it be to love someone:

who winds metres of sellotape around his body and must be rescued from it?
who tries to flag down an auto secretly while we wait for the valet to bring our car?
whose idea of hiding in a game of hide-n-seek is getting down on all fours in the middle of the room and covering his face with his hands?

who thinks it's incredibly hip to have a handkerchief folded in a triangle pinned to his shirt to wipe snot from his nose?

who believes I invented the alphabet, numbers, taxonomy of plants and animals, names for natural phenomena and every other discipline of knowledge known to a four-year-old?

who goes berserk with happiness and excitement when I enter the room for no other reason than that I entered the room?

Before Advaith, I did not know that I could feel such tenderness. That I could be besotted by someone's chubby hands and round cheeks, by the small Os that his mouth makes in wonderment or the black liquidness of his trusting eyes. That I could miss someone so achingly, especially one who has crowded me out of my own life. That someone quite literally born yesterday could have such sway on my state of mind and the lens with which I view the world. And while there are any number of ways in which our lives and families can be imagined, with or without children, I am glad I made this call. In retrospect, I can say it feels utterly worthwhile.

Because this is a love unlike any other that I have experienced. A love bigger than me and my ego, insecurities, limitations and preoccupations. A love so potent that it can make bruises, aches and ailments disappear. A love so vulnerable that it cannot withstand a single degree of separation. A love so light and nimble that it is expressed in crayons and glitter glue, oversized letters of the alphabet and muddy hands and feet. A love so strong and heavy that no cards, poems or letters can contain it. A love so in-the-moment that it exults in train rides, ice-cream cones, merry-go-rounds and superhero costumes. A love so abiding that it seeks me out amidst all the thrills and attractions of this world. And what's life without a little love?

Epilogue

'No man ever steps in the same river twice, for it's not the same river and he's not the same man.'—Heraclitus

Looking back now, I don't feel a sense of accomplishment or triumph in having had a child. I don't have the swagger of a warrior who has waged a tenacious battle and emerged victorious. Mostly, what I have is a feeling of having survived. The feeling of having made it by the skin of my teeth. In many ways I feel 'lucky'—a blend of relief, incredulity and thankfulness for the exceptional circumstances that brought me to motherhood.

When I was knee-deep in infertility, I was at pains to explain its purpose in my life. Was it a penalty for past karma? Was it the universe trying to hand out a life lesson? Why was I at the receiving end of this suffering? Now, after acquiring the perspective that distance and time grant, I am convinced there was nothing personal about it. It was not a morality tale and I was not singled out to be schooled by infertility. It was a stray encounter, a random occurrence like the conditions of our birth and death, complicated by a multitude of determinants such as lifestyle, partner, age, genes and physiology. This thinking has freed me to a certain degree from the guilt and self-blame I struggled with. It's not a blot on my past, a red mark in my report card. On the contrary, it was a rich, intense and compelling journey, even though I didn't consider it so then. And I happened to emerge with a baby at the other end.

Even if the universe had not purposely planned to mould and shape me through infertility, the manner in which I received this ordeal gave me an opportunity to expand, both in belly and mind. A number of notions I carried close to my chest crumbled under its weight. For instance, my cocksure faith in medicine. Medicine brought the baby into our lives, or at least created the conditions for it to be born. But it was not a straight input-in-output-out scenario. There were many variables, like implantation, that were beyond our control. I could have just as easily ended up at the wrong end of the success ratio statistics, and medicine would have just shrugged its shoulders and said 'bad luck'. My belief in medicine had to be caveated; there were limits to its powers.

I developed a new reverence for my body, for the physical and chemical processes animating it, the elaborate and intricate dance of reproduction that takes place beyond human scrutiny or even understanding. I was so used to neglecting my body and yet enjoying the rewards of good health. Until then, self-care was a superficial affair, mostly translated as staying thin. In the last IVF cycle that led to the birth of my son, I consciously avoided caffeine, cut down my sugar intake, drank plenty of fluids and slowed down to enjoy who I was and where I was. During the fifteen-day interval between the embryo transfer and the home pregnancy test, I started viewing my body with compassion rather than with hostility and impatience at its non-performance. When I changed my stance, my body returned the love.

I spent a long time erecting fences against what I saw as unnatural or invasive or just painful. The resistance came not just from the need to protect myself but was rooted in denial about my infertility. In my script of the perfect life there was no space to accommodate infertility. It was a bad dream and would be over soon. I waited months before seeking help, hoping that I could avoid the stigma of going to a fertility clinic. I was positive that IUI would work and I could pretend it was 'natural'. I hoped that once pregnant I would never miscarry because the heartache would be too much to bear. But I learnt that unless you accept what you are undergoing, you can't get past it. I had to stand my ground, look that beast in the eye and brace myself for the fight. Anticipating immunity from loss and pain only left me unprepared. Acceptance of my imperfect reality, acceptance of the possibility of failure and the possibility that 'success' might never come gave me the strength and equanimity to go back and keep submitting myself to the vagaries of reproductive science.

I now know intimately several women who have experienced infertility. Some of us have conceived without any intervention, some through IUI or IVF, some have adopted, while some of us are yet to come to the end of our stories. When I meet someone who is in the same plight as I once was, I feel the need to jump in and share my story. To deliver a pep talk and offer exclusive takeaways from my own encounter. Telling them to keep at it. That it will happen someday. I feel deeply the trauma these women are going through and want nothing more than for them to succeed. Yet, I am aware that some of us will not have a happy resolution, or at least not the one we have fantasized about. To say it's happened for me so it will happen for you too seems facile. I am reminded of a talk I heard on TV once. You may do everything in your capacity to ensure you have a healthy body and mind, but you cannot stubbornly insist you must never fall ill. That is the way of life. Let the river run its course.

In the meantime, what I can offer is my compassion, support and solidarity. Sister, my ears and shoulders are all yours.

Acknowledgements

I am indebted to:
Pooja Hiranandani—for her magnanimity and friendship, for offering to read and edit the first draft at a time of great turbulence in her own life.

Bhawani Cheerath—for her time and generosity, for reading and reviewing early drafts several times.

Nilanjan P. Choudhury—for his help, counsel and camaraderie, for being the first champion of this book when it didn't seem like it had a future.

Aswana Mathew-Srinivasraghavan—for forcing me to rewrite chapters that I thought were done and dusted, for being the biggest cheerleader of this book and its author.

Reshmi Mitra, Meera Nair, Nadika Nadja, Aniruddha Malpani and Sreeparna Chattopadhyay—for their thoughtful feedback and invaluable support at various points during this journey.

Maya Jayapal—for welcoming me with open arms into her life, for gently nudging me in the right direction whenever

I have sought guidance, for extending her warmth and compassion at all times.

Jayapriya Vasudevan—for throwing her weight behind this manuscript, for sharing her wisdom in times of doubt, for being the agent a debut author can only dream of.

Gurveen Chadha—for believing in this story, for embracing it with remarkable empathy and sensitivity, and for letting me tell it the way I wanted to.

Shreya Chakravertty and Kripa Raman—for their meticulous and thorough work as copy editors, for closing gaps, tying loose ends and catching inconsistencies.

Devangana Dash—for the splendid work on the book cover.

Dr M, Dr U and J—for staying with me resolutely on a long and difficult journey.

Rama Murthy Sripada and Anusha Shetty—for being the people I can always count on.

Amma, Achan, Remya and Vikram—for the security and comfort of family.

Amma and Ammamma—for being the centre and certainty of my universe.

Gopal and Archana—for allowing me to represent parts of their life. Gopal—for being the receptacle into which I poured this story, chapter by chapter, weekend after weekend, for being my oldest friend and the only cool head in the family.

Ranjith—for everything. For knowing when to fade into the background and when to take centrestage, when to be saviour and when just an observer, for the perfect balance between affection and respect, allowing solitude and extending solidarity.

Advaith—for the love, for the love I didn't know existed until you arrived.

References

1. American Pregnancy Association, 'What Is HCG?', https://americanpregnancy.org/while-pregnant/hcg-levels/, accessed in August 2020.

2. American Pregnancy Association, 'Early Fetal Development', https://americanpregnancy.org/pregnancy-complications/early-fetal-development, accessed in August 2020.

3. Apollo Fertility, 'How Many Eggs Is a Woman Born with', https://www.apollofertility.com/blog/fertility/how-many-eggs-is-a-woman-born-with, accessed in August 2020.

4. Belle Boggs, *The Art of Waiting* (Graywolf Press, 2016).

5. Krissi Danielson, 'Crown Rump Length (CRL) on Ultrasounds', Verywell Family, https://www.verywellfamily.com/crown-rump-length-crl-2371608, last updated on 2 February 2020.

6. Krissi Danielson, 'Why hCG Doubling Times Are Important in Early Pregnancy', Verywell Family, https://www.verywellfamily.com/normal-hcg-doubling-times-

240 REFERENCES

in-early-pregnancy-2371282, last updated on 10 January 2020.

7. Catherine Donaldson-Evans, 'Subchorionic Bleeding during Pregnancy', What to Expect, https://www.whattoexpect.com/pregnancy/pregnancy-health/complications/subchorionic-bleeding.aspx, reviewed on 28 October 2019.

8. Sian Ferguson, 'What Is Diminished Ovarian Reserve and What Can You Do about It?', Healthline Parenthood, https://www.healthline.com/health/diminished-ovarian-reserve#treatment, reviewed on 26 February 2019.

9. FertilitySmarts, 'Trilaminar endometrium', https://www.fertilitysmarts.com/definition/2102/trilaminar-endometrium, last updated on 8 April 2020.

10. FertilitySmarts, 'Blastocyst', https://www.fertilitysmarts.com/definition/230/blastocyst, last updated on 17 April 2020.

11. Focus on Reproduction, 'A Cut-off for Endometrial Thickness: Findings from the Largest Cohort Study', 30 October 2018, https://www.focusonreproduction.eu/article/News-in-Reproduction-endometrium.

12. Amos Grünebaum, 'Crown Rump Length Chart: Fetal Ultrasound Measurements', BabyMed, https://www.babymed.com/fetus-crown-rump-length-crl-measurements-ultrasound, last updated on 18 January 2019.

13. Amos Grünebaum, 'In-Vitro Fertilization (IVF): What Is It?', BabyMed, https://www.babymed.com/ivf/what-is-ivf-in-vitro-fertilization, last updated on 29 June 2020.

14. Rachel Gurevich, 'How Ovarian and Antral Follicles Relate to Fertility', Verywell Family, https://www.

verywellfamily.com/follicle-female-reproductive-system-1960072, reviewed on 20 July 2020.

15. M.S. Kamath, R. Kirubakaran, S. Sunkara, 'Use of granulocyte-colony stimulating factor during in vitro fertilisation treatment', Cochrane, 24 January 2020, https://www.cochrane.org/CD013226/MENSTR_use-granulocyte-colony-stimulating-factor-during-vitro-fertilisation-treatment.

16. Gideon Koren, et al., 'The Protective Effects of Nausea and Vomiting of Pregnancy against Adverse Fetal Outcome—a Systematic Review', *Reproductive Toxicology* vol. 47 (2014): pp. 77–80, https://doi:10.1016/j.reprotox.2014.05.012.

17. Paul C. Magarelli, 'IUI Success Rates', CNY Fertility, https://www.cnyfertility.com/iui-success-rates/, last updated on 8 September 2020.

18. Aniruddha Malpani, 'Treating a Thin Endometrial Lining', Malpani Infertility Clinic, https://www.drmalpani.com/knowledge-center/articles/thin-endometrial-lining, accessed in August 2020.

19. Aniruddha Malpani, 'Putting the Myth of Bed Rest after IVF to Rest', https://blog.drmalpani.com/2008/04/putting-myth-of-bed-rest-after-ivf-to.html, accessed in August 2020.

20. Aniruddha Malpani, 'What Is Beta HCG Test, Interpretations of Beta HCG Levels in Pregnancy', Malpani Infertility Clinic, https://www.drmalpani.com/knowledge-center/articles/betahcglevels, accessed in August 2020.

21. Ashley Marcin, 'What Is Ovulation? 16 Things to Know about Your Menstrual Cycle', Healthline Parenthood,

https://www.healthline.com/health/womens-health/ what-is-ovulation, accessed on 10 July 2018.

22. Mayo Clinic, 'Miscarriage', https://www.mayoclinic. org/diseases-conditions/pregnancy-loss-miscarriage/ symptoms-causes/syc-20354298, accessed in August 2020.

23. Mayo Clinic, 'Ovarian Hyperstimulation Syndrome', https://www.mayoclinic.org/diseases-conditions/ ovarian-hyperstimulation-syndrome-ohss/symptoms- causes/syc-20354697, accessed in August 2020.

24. Eric R. Olson, 'Why Are 250 Million Sperm Cells Released during Sex?', Livescience, 24 January 2013, https://www. livescience.com/32437-why-are-250-million-sperm- cells-released-during-sex.html.

25. Stephanie Pildner von Steinburg, Anne-Laure Boulesteix, Christian Lederer, et al., 'What Is the "Normal" Fetal Heart Rate?', *PeerJ* (2013): 1:e82, https://doi.org/10.7717/ peerj.82.

26. Andrea Rodrigo, Sara Salgado, Valeria Sotelo and Sandra Fernandez, 'The Intrauterine Insemination (IUI) Process Step by Step', inviTRA, https://www.invitra.com/en/ artificial-insemination-process, last updated on 1 August 2019.

27. Edurne Martinez Sanz, Gorka Barrenetxea Ziarrusta, Juan José Espinós Gómez, María Eugenia Ballesteros Moffa, Rebeca Reus and Romina Packan, 'How Does the Frozen Embryo Transfer (FET) Procedure Work?', inviTRA, https://www.invitra.com/en/frozen-embryo-transfer/, last updated on 6 January 2020.

28. Sanchita Sharma and Anonna Dutt, '40 Years of IVF: See How Fertility Tech Has Changed the World, and

India', *Hindustan Times*, 21 July 2018, https://www.hindustantimes.com/india-news/40-years-of-ivf-see-how-fertility-tech-has-changed-the-world-and-india/story-ow9SKhft9Z9ZUJXo9jTtvO.html.

29. Ultrasoundpaedia, 'First Trimester Ultrasound—Normal', https://www.ultrasoundpaedia.com/normal-1sttrimester, accessed in August 2020.

30. WebMD, 'Bleeding during Pregnancy', https://www.webmd.com/baby/guide/bleeding-during-pregnancy#1, accessed in August 2020.